BEYOND TECHNIQUE IN SOLUTION-FOCUSED THERAPY

The Guilford Family Therapy Series

Michael P. Nichols, Series Editor

Recent Volumes

Beyond Technique in Solution-Focused Therapy

Working with Emotions and the Therapeutic Relationship

Eve Lipchik

Foreword by Wendel A. Ray

THE GUILFORD PRESS
New York   London

© 2002 The Guilford Press
A Division of Guilford Publications, Inc.
72 Spring Street, New York, NY 10012
www.guilford.com

Printed in the United States of America

This book is printed on acid-free paper.

Last digit is print number: 9   8   7   6   5   4   3   2   1

Library of Congress Cataloging-in-Publication Data

Lipchik, Eve.
  Beyond technique in solution-focused therapy : working with emotions
and the therapeutic relationship / by Eve Lipchik.
       p. cm. — (The Guilford family therapy series)
Includes biographical references and index.
  ISBN 1-57230-764-1
  1. Solution-focused therapy. I. Title. II. Series.
RC489.S65 L565 2002
616.89′14—dc21   2002005515

To Elliot,
who invented consideration and generosity

About the Author

Eve Lipchik, MSW, a member of the American Family Therapy Academy and a certified member and approved supervisor of the American Association for Marriage and Family Therapy, cofounded ICF Consultants, Incorporated, in Milwaukee, Wisconsin, in 1988. From 1980 until 1988, Ms. Lipchik was a core member of the Brief Family Therapy Center in Milwaukee, where she participated in the development of solution-focused therapy. In addition to her private practice, she teaches, consults, and lectures both nationally and internationally. She is the editor of *Interviewing* and has been published in numerous books and journals, including the *Psychotherapy Networker*, the *Journal of Systemic Therapies*, and *Family Process*.

Foreword

It would be surprising if Eve Lipchik remembered meeting a particular one of the countless therapists she has taught, but I clearly recall my first experience with her, in May 1983, during an intensive training program at the Brief Family Therapy Center. The highlight of this weeklong immersion in the work of Steve de Shazer, Insoo Berg, and their team was an afternoon spent talking with and watching Eve work. So impressive was her grasp of theory, skill as a teacher, and remarkable therapeutic ability that I began following her work. Over the years I have read Eve's contributions to the brief family therapy and solution-focused literatures and, whenever the opportunity presented itself, attended her teaching seminars and workshops, always coming away feeling stimulated by the profound implications of her thinking and by her ability to translate the most complex ideas into down-to-earth, clinical applications.

Beginning with an insider's history of the development of solution-focused therapy (SFT), readers are presented with a remarkably clear explication of SFT theory and practice. What comes out is the author's journey from discomfort with the pat answers she felt emerging in more naive understandings of SFT to an unfolding of her own brand of SFT, which I would describe as *emotion-centered* solution-focused brief therapy.

A major contribution of this volume is the reintroduction of theory into the practice of therapy, especially the author's reintegration of essential conceptions from interpersonally oriented psychotherapies. She offers readers' tenets that are absolutely fundamental to the *doing* of effective, efficient, and *humanistic* brief therapy.

In an era that ignores the past and, in a perpetual search for ever more simple and uncomplicated answers to complex questions, tends to overvalue anything presented as "new," Eve has accomplished a complete reversal: She explores and embraces the "new" while investigating and revitalizing elements of existing knowledge. Drawing from the seminal work of Harry Stack Sullivan, Gregory Bateson, Don D. Jackson, Milton Erickson, Jay Haley, John Weakland, Richard Fisch, Paul Watzlawick, and others, she outlines then breathes life into theoretical conceptions that are the cornerstones of both the brief therapy model developed at the Mental Research Institute and SFT.

Building on this infrastructure, Eve also incorporates ideas from a broad range of disciplines such as biology, linguistics, cybernetics, constructionism, anthropology, and social constructivism. Her crystal-clear interpretations of the sophisticated contributions of Maturana and Varela are especially valuable and timely.

An example is in order. Thanks to Eve's effort, a marvelously useful merging of the fresh and new with the time-proven can be seen by juxtaposing Maturana's definition of love with that of Harry Stack Sullivan. According to one reference cited by Eve, for Maturana, love is behavior that "allows the other to arise as a legitimate other in coexistence with oneself" and "opens up the possibility of seeing and hearing that other." Sullivan phrases it this way: "When the satisfaction or security of another person becomes as significant to one as one's own satisfaction and security, then a state of love exists" (1953a, pp. 42–43). In recent times the world of psychotherapy, in its tendency to understand by means of lineal causal logic and perpetuation of a Cartesian dualistic separation of mind and body, has downplayed the vital part human relations play in mental health, particularly such sticky ones as love. And yet readers who do not appreciate the relevance of such basic emotions in understanding human distress and the practice of psychotherapy might as well pull down their ears and keep dozing because we are simply not on the same wavelength.[1]

Yet another advancement pioneered by Eve Lipchik is the exploration of inquiry as perturbation or, in my language, intervention. This is one of the most significant advances to have occurred in the field of therapy and, to my knowledge, only Eve Lipchik, Gianfranco Cecchin, and Richard Fisch, each working independently, are explicitly researching, practicing, and honing this phenomenal breakthrough.

---

[1]Apologies and deference to Jackson (1963) for first introducing this vivid phrasing.

Inquiry as intervention and the linking of essential premises developed in the past with current cutting-edge thinking are major contributions made in this important book, but from my point of view by far not the most significant. In synthesizing these broad areas and fleshing out the logic and nuances of her approach, Eve makes a groundbreaking contribution to clinical practice: reintroduction of human emotion into the practice of brief therapy (I say reintroduction because emotion was central in the work of such early pioneers as Harry Stack Sullivan, Don D. Jackson, and Milton Erickson).

In a lecture to residents given at the Washington School of Psychiatry shortly before his death in 1949, Harry Stack Sullivan made the following prediction:

> The same things that make psychiatry slippery for others make it slippery for me; it is awfully easy to be deceived. But a much more practical psychotherapy seems to be possible when one seeks to find the basic vulnerabilities to anxiety in interpersonal relations, rather than to deal [only] with symptoms called out by anxiety or to avoid anxiety. (1953b, p. 11)

By daring to tackle distressing emotions as distinctly anxiety-evoked adaptations to unique interpersonal phenomena, Eve Lipchik, in this skillfully written and pragmatic volume, has moved the field another vital step further along toward the fulfillment of Sullivan's prophecy.

WENDEL A. RAY, PhD
Director, Mental Research Institute, Palo Alto, California
Professor of Family Therapy, University of Louisiana–Monroe

Preface

Solution-focused therapy (SFT) has become well established as a strength-based and brief therapy model. However, neither its appeal to managed care nor reports about its efficacy have been able to quell doubts about its ability to promote permanent change or address clients' emotional needs. The intentions of this book are to demonstrate a way of thinking about and practicing SFT that negates these doubts and demonstrates its depth and breadth.

SFT did not arise de novo. It is founded on the work of Gregory Bateson, Milton Erickson, Don Jackson, John Weakland, Jay Haley, Paul Watzlawick, and others who are credited with developing the systemic paradigm. It is the end result of the efforts of a group of people who sat around at the Brief Family Therapy Center in Milwaukee almost a quarter of a century ago and energized each other with their enthusiasm for new ideas about how people change. The core of this group consisted of Steve de Shazer, Insoo Berg, Jim Derks, Elam Nunnally, Marilyn LaCourt, and myself. As time went on the group was nourished by students who became colleagues, including John Walter, Jane Peller, Alex Molnar, Kate Kowalski, and Michele Weiner-Davis, and by academicians such as Gale Miller and Wally Gingerich. What started out as a model called Brief Family Therapy evolved into SFT. Gradually some members of the group left and others joined. I left in 1988, and started ICF Consultants in Milwaukee with Marilyn Bonjean. I think it is fair to say that everyone who ever participated in the conversations at the Brief Family Therapy Center made a contribution, and that everyone gained from the experience. The prolific solution-focused literature reflects the wealth and diversity of their experience.

Today, SFT is world famous but often misunderstood, and even trivialized. In my opinion, this is the result of an overemphasis on the techniques and the loss of a theoretical framework. Techniques applied out of context can have dramatic short-term results that do not make much difference in the long run.

The theory and practice of SFT proposed here restores an interactional context to the techniques based on what therapists at the Mental Research Institute refer to as "positioning themselves" in relation to clients or what therapists at the Brief Family Therapy Center called "cooperating with how clients cooperate." This concept can still be considered relevant to a practice informed by constructivism if language is thought of as mutually influenced behavior.

To some extent I developed my present clinical approach in reaction to minimalism and the postmodern intellectualization of therapy. Although I, too, have always aspired to elegant, well-targeted interventions, I have come to believe they are most likely to succeed in the context of a trusting therapist–client relationship. This belief is supported by a research study conducted by David Kiser at the Brief Family Therapy Center in 1988, which indicated that clients who came for a greater number of sessions reported higher rates of success.

By the same token, I am in full agreement with the postmodern emphasis on highly individualized treatment, though I have been concerned about the general lack of guidelines for practice, supervision, and teaching.

Finally, I have not been able to reconcile myself with isolating language from the living human systems we are. This has stimulated an interest in physiological aspects of language and emotion.

My efforts to integrate some of my conflicting ideas have been influenced by Harry Stack Sullivan's theory of interpersonal psychiatry, and more recently by Maturana and Varela's theory of cognition, and developments in neuroscientific research.

Emotions have always been a subject non grata in SFT. Like my colleagues, I avoided "emotion talk" religiously for some years before I noticed that addressing emotions often enables clients who feel stuck to move forward more easily. At the same time, my interest in the therapist–client relationship kept bringing the positive effects of talking with clients about their feelings into relief.

Teaching, supervising, consulting, and presenting workshops have challenged me to understand my own thinking in order to help others develop theirs. It also highlighted the importance of relationship, regardless of its purpose. This book therefore stresses the importance of thera-pists as people in relation to their clients and strives to answer the ques-tion of how we can both use, and keep separate, our personal and professional selves to benefit clients.

Our customary approach to training at the Brief Family Therapy Center was to throw trainees into the ring with clients, equipped only with a few basic questions. We believed that support from the supervisor and team behind the mirror would allay their anxiety and ensure good quality of service for the clients. Yet, many clients did not return after their initial sessions. What we thought was a well-constructed message composed by the supervisor and team apparently did not compensate for an interview that left clients dissatisfied. What consequently proved to work better for the clients was their perception that someone was listen-ing to them and trying to understand what they were trying to communi-cate. This approach also benefited the beginning therapists because it made them less likely to use techniques out of context.

Two personal experiences have been instrumental in shaping the ideas in this book. One was an occasion when John Weakland visited the Brief Family Therapy Center in the late 1980s. He came periodically to conduct workshops in Milwaukee, or to consult with our team. After one of these workshops, during which he had interviewed clients in front of the mirror, he asked whether we would like to see a videotape he had brought along of a session he did in Palo Alto. Of course we wanted to. We could never get enough of watching "the Master" work. All I recall now was that the clients were elderly and the problem concerned some issues with their children, but I have not forgotten the extent of my sur-prise. Up to that point I would have described John's manner of inter-viewing as minimalist. However, on this tape he responded more, and attended to the clients' feelings in a deliberate and gentle manner. He did not take a break to formulate a message at the end of the session yet came up with a sensitive and brilliant intervention with barely a pause to think. When we questioned him about this difference in style, he said this was a session he had conducted in his private practice, where he could "just do therapy." At the Mental Research Institute Clinic, or at workshops, he felt he had to demonstrate the brief model. While inter-views deliberately stripped of extraneous niceties might highlight the Mental Research Institute techniques better, I felt that the taped inter-view was a much better demonstration of the Mental Research Institute model. It stimulated me to think about how to integrate the technical and humanistic aspects into SFT.

The second experience occurred in 1996, in Heidelberg, Germany, at a conference titled "Science/Fiction: Fundamentalism and Arbitrariness in Science and Therapy," organized by the Heidelberg Institute for Systemic Research and the International Association for Systemic Therapy. Humberto Maturana was the plenary speaker. He pointed out that it is an emotion he romantically calls "love" that makes us human. This is the behavior that makes us accept another human being "as a legitimate other in existence with ourselves" and therefore allows us to see and hear that other person for who he or she is. He went on to say that this is "the ground in which reflection can take place, the work of the therapist can take place, and the ground in which the problems of human relations are solved." This statement crystallized the idea for me that for the sake of our clients we should think of ourselves first as human beings, second as therapists, and only last as therapists who practice a particular model.

A primary goal of this book is to provide answers to the questions most frequently asked by solution-focused therapists at all levels of experience, such as "How do I know I am being solution-focused?"; "How can I be where the client is and focus on positives at the same time?"; "What do I respond to, and what do I ignore?"; "Can I do SFT with long-term clients?" The material is arranged to provide a logical way for clinicians to think about how the solution-focused assumptions guide the decision-making process. Descriptions of how to guide the therapist–client relationship, how to clarify the problem to define goals that lead to solutions, and how to formulate the summation message and tailor-make fitting suggestions are provided. These interactions between therapist and client are considered from both perspectives so clinicians can develop an awareness of their own process in relation to clients, and its effects. The use of emotions is interwoven throughout the book as well as treated in a separate chapter. Applications to couples, families, involuntary clients, and crisis work is also included.

This is primarily a clinical book. Therefore, it contains a lot of annotated case material that is deliberately longer and more detailed in the earlier chapters than later, when the readers will have a better understanding of the basic principles.

Acknowledgments

This book would never have been written without the wonderful introduction I received to the mental health field when I worked for the Primary Mental Health Project in Rochester, New York. I want to start by thanking everyone there, in particular Ellie Eksten, a truly devoted supervisor. My positive experience at the Project was continued as a graduate student at the University of Rochester under the supervision of Helen Kristal. Thank you, Helen, for making me toe the line and setting high standards for my work! This is equally true for John Jendusa, my field placement instructor at the University of Wisconsin in Milwaukee. These three fine professionals taught me that clinical supervisors have an enormous responsibility toward their supervisees.

I am also deeply grateful for the opportunity to have participated in the development of the theory and practice of SFT at the Brief Family Therapy Center. It has been one of the most transforming experiences in my life.

I want to thank Sharon Stoffel and Pat O'Hearn for meeting with me for consultation so faithfully over the years. They are role models for the conscientious practitioner and their work has enriched me greatly. Over the past decade I have had the privilege of teaching SFT to the staff of community agencies such as Jewish Family Service, Midwest Clinical Services, and St. Aemilian/Lakeside. This gave me the opportunity to work with people of different theoretical orientations over long periods. I thank all of them for challenging me to connect my thinking to theirs in a way that will be useful for them. Many of the ideas in this book were inspired by their questions and thoughtful replies.

A word of thanks to Michelle Wilson, Andrew Turnell, and Steve Edwards at the Centrecare Family Agency in Perth, Australia, for giving me the opportunity to apply solution-focused work at the other end of the globe. Meeting with their colleagues and clients, particularly with members of the Aboriginal culture, was truly a growth experience.

The direct inspiration for this book came from 9 days of intensive training conducted at the Institute for Marriage and Family Therapy in Vienna, Austria, in the summer of 1997. The interdisciplinary participants were committed practitioners, well versed in systemic and constructivist thinking. Most of them had had previous training in SFT. When we first met, we developed a set of questions that represented the goals for the training. These questions turned out to encompass the issues with which most practitioners struggle. The idea for a book that would answer the questions occurred to me during that time. I want to thank Joachim Hinsch, the director, for the opportunity to conduct that training, as well as Corina Alhlers, Hedi Wagner, Andrea Brandl-Nebehay, and all the extraordinarily thoughtful participants.

Once I began to write this book my business partner—and friend—Marilyn Bonjean supported me even more than usual. I thank her for her perfect partnership. Words are also insufficient to express my appeciation to Mark Becker, Brett Brasher, Jim Derks, Marilyn LaCourt, and Jane Volkman for their invaluable help throughout the entire process. They generously took time from their busy schedules to provide caring, challenging, and judicious editorial comments, not to mention emotional support. I am equally grateful to Mike Nichols for his careful editing. Thanks also go to Gillian Denavit, a serious student of SFT, but one who is still getting her feet wet clinically, for providing me with the perspective of the novice. Her questions and comments were helpful. A special word of appreciation to Kate Kowalski for her friendship, support, and editorial comments.

Last, but far from least, I want to thank my husband, our children, and their partners for their loving support, and our grandchildren for their smiles and kisses that energized me all the way.

Contents

BEYOND TECHNIQUE IN
SOLUTION-FOCUSED THERAPY

Part I

Theory and Practice

A Theory of
Solution-Focused Therapy

A solution-focused therapist felt stuck with a case and asked for help. He had had four sessions with John, a 46-year-old married attorney, with two teenage daughters, but after an initial report of improvement the solution seemed unclear. John had described his reason for coming to therapy as "being at the end of my rope in dealing with my widowed father." His brother-in-law, a physician, had suggested he ask his doctor for some medication, but John considered medicine a crutch.

John appeared extremely agitated during the first session. He was flushed, picked at one of his cuticles constantly, and spoke so rapidly that he had to stop and catch his breath at times. He related that his mother had died 5 months ago at age 75, leaving his 78-year-old father alone after 51 years of marriage.

John was one of four siblings, and the only one who lived in the same city as the parents. Since his mother's death, John and his family had made a special effort to be supportive to his father. At first this effort was appreciated, but as time went on his father became increasingly hostile and hard to satisfy. John's wife had urged John not to take his father's behavior so personally, but John was not able to avoid such feelings. The final straw had been when his father had refused to speak to him while on a visit to John's sister because "he didn't want to hear my voice." Since then, John had been unable to sleep or concentrate on his work.

John perceived that his relationship with his parents prior to his mother's death had been agreeable. He and his family saw John's parents at least once a week and spent all major holidays and birthdays with them. Although the father had always expressed criticism more than praise, his mother's warm, nurturing ways had more than made up for it.

When the therapist had attempted to get John to define his problem and goals in behavioral terms, the best John could do was to say he wanted to learn to cope with his father's ways so he could be a good son. He recognized that he could not change an old man. He described his father's behavior toward him as "eating away my insides." He would know he was better when "his father's words would go in one ear and out another." John was unable to answer how his own behavior would change when that began to occur. The therapist had asked an exception question in relation to that goal: "Are there times when you already let your father's words go in one ear and out another?" John could think of only one example, shortly after his mother died, when he had felt very sorry for his father. The therapist tried to build on that exception by asking, "What was different at those times? What would you have to do now to make that happen, even a little bit?", but John was unable to answer.

The therapist then turned to another technique, the miracle question. "If you go to bed tonight and a miracle happens while you are asleep, and when you wake up in the morning your problem is solved, how will things be different?" John had answered that he would ignore the behavior. "Does that happen already at times?" the therapist asked. Not at present, said John. "What will you have to do to make that happen? Is there anything someone else could do to make that happen?" John said he felt he had no control at present to change anything.

At the end of the first session the therapist had composed an intervention message which complimented John for his desire to learn to cope with his father's behavior and for wanting to be a good son. It expressed empathy with John's difficult position, having to mourn his mother at the same time that he had to deal with his father's rejecting ways. The intensity of John's reaction was reframed as an unusually strong commitment to family. The therapist had also designed a task for John to give him a sense of control again. The task suggested that John give himself a break from being in touch with his father for 3 days as his father was being cared for by his sister. If, during that time, he ever felt comfortable about calling and wanted to do it to make himself feel good rather than to please his father, he could do so. However, if he felt ambivalent about calling, he was to remind himself that he did not have to make that decision until the fourth day. On the fourth day he was to call but talk only to his sister and to tell her to tell his father he called to inquire about him.

When John returned a week later the therapist measured change by asking a scaling question: "On a scale from 1 to 10, with 10 being that you are as stressed as you can be, and 1 being that you are totally relaxed, where would you say you are today?" (de Shazer, 1991a, p. 148). John reported that his stress level had decreased from a 10 to a 7. He had chosen to call his father on the second day and had not felt as uncomfortable as he expected to even though his father had been short and unfriendly. Since then he had made one more call and also tolerated it better.

During the second session the therapist and John worked on reinforcing this increased comfort and tolerance John had described by discussing "What will have to happen for more of that to happen? What could you do? What could others do to help you?" The therapist also looked for resources from the past that could help John in the present situation by asking, "How have you dealt successfully with stressful personal relationships in the past?" At the end of the session the therapist complimented John on having gained some control in relation to his father and told him to continue doing what he had been doing.

During the third session John reported that his father had returned home. John had picked him up at the airport, and his father had immediately criticized John for not having been clear whether he would meet him at the gate or at the baggage claim. Since then there had been several difficult phone conversations that led John to feel his stress level was an 8 on a scale of 10 again. John repeated that he wanted to find a solution without medication.

In an effort to stay away from the problem and look toward a solution the therapist had revisited the exception that occurred between the first and second session. What was different then? John thought it might have been the fact that his father was in another city. It made him feel less responsible when his father was with his sister. At the end of the session John was given the task to pretend his father is in another city when he speaks with him over the phone. When he met with him in person he was to imagine his sister, or his brother in the room, as well. John did not report any improvement as a result of this task and appeared discouraged about his lack of progress.

Why was this case not progressing? The therapist was clearly doing solution-focused therapy (hereafter SFT) as it is generally understood. He had the client describe the problem and define a goal in behavioral terms.

Once John had described his problem, the therapist had used the exception question (de Shazer, 1985; Lipchik, 1988a), and the miracle question (de Shazer, 1988; Friedman, 1993; Lipchik, 1988a; Nau & Shilts, 2000). At one point, when the therapist was not getting any useful responses from John he had asked the coping question (Lipchik, 1988a): "How come things aren't worse? What have you done to keep things from getting worse?" This question often produces some strengths clients can build on, but it had not helped in this situation. The therapist had used the scaling question (de Shazer, 1991a) to measure change.

At the end of the sessions the therapist had offered thoughtful intervention messages and tasks that built on positives and made use of the client's way of experiencing the world, such as his need for control and his particular use of language. Why didn't any of these techniques lead to a solution for the client?

The answer is simple: SFT is more than the trademark techniques it is known for. It is a sophisticated therapeutic model that has been applied to a variety of situations such as adoption (Shaffer & Lindstrom, 1989), aging (Bonjean, 1989, 1996; Dahl, Bathel, & Carreon, 2000), alcohol abuse (Berg & Miller, 1992; Brasher, Campbell, & Moen, 1993), child protection services (Berg & Kelly, 2000; Turnell & Edwards, 1999), domestic violence (Lipchik, 1991; Lipchik & Kubicki, 1996; Lipchik, Sirles, & Kubicki, 1997; Tucker, Stith, Howell, McCollum, & Rosen, 2000), family-based services (Berg, 1994), multiple personality disorder (Barker & Herlache, 1997), physically impaired clients (Ahlers, 1992), residential treatment (Booker & Blymer, 1994; Durrant, 1993), sexual abuse (Dolan, 1991; Kowalski, 1987), school problems (Durrant, 1995; Kral, 1992; Metcalf, 1995; Molnar & Lindquist, 1989; Murphy, 1996), spirituality (Simon, 1996), children (Selekman, 1997), and more. SFT takes time and experience to master, just like any other therapeutic approach.

Perhaps SFT has been misunderstood because it was conceived as a minimalist way of intervening, a pragmatic way of problem solving (de Shazer, 1982, 1985, 1988, 1991a, 1994). Minimalism may have been interpreted to mean that all the therapist needs to do is to ask questions. Of course, that was never intended. At the Brief Family Therapy Center the prerequisite for trainees was a master's degree in a mental health discipline and 2 years of clinical experience. We expected people who were going to learn our model to be skilled in establishing and maintaining a therapeutic alliance. Unfortunately, we did not emphasize that in the literature but concentrated on describing the new ideas. I never realized that misunderstanding until much later, when I showed a videotape at a seminar to demonstrate the use of questions as interventions. After watching for a few minutes a well-known colleague heaved a sigh of relief and said, "Oh, you contextualize those questions."

Although minimalism may have been misunderstood in practice, it did have a theoretical base and assumptions that offered guidelines beside questions. However, under the influence of postmodernism, theory was dismissed as antithetical to truly individualized treatment (Held, 1996, 2000). This new direction reduced SFT to "nothing but language"(de Shazer, 1994; Miller & de Shazer, 1998), another description that is open to misinterpretation. Language in postmodern theory is generally thought of in the broad sense

> as located in the consensual behavioral interactions between persons, not inside "the mind" of either. Rather than a vehicle that carries abstract communication back and forth between individual minds, it is a coordination of bodily states within members of a social group that preserves the structural integrity of both the social group and that of each group member. (Griffith & Griffith, 1994, p. 312)

Language is not intended to mean only the words people speak. However, even the broad description of language fails to guide therapists in using language to help clients find solutions. No wonder the solution-focused questions appear so attractive! They offer something concrete with which to work. The problem is that emphasis on form over substance usually does not give the desired results (Cecchin, Lane, & Ray, 1992).

The case of John, described previously, illustrates my point. The therapist used the basic techniques in the first session and had some positive results. When these changes were not sustained after the second session, the therapist continued to follow what he understood to be the right solution-focused direction. He tried scaling and coping questions to no avail.

To help this therapist get unstuck in consultation he was asked to think, "What is going on between John and me that might be causing this impasse?" He answered, "I am asking questions and giving tasks that are not making a difference. I have to do something different." However, he was perplexed about what that might be, given that he had used all the right techniques.

The next suggestion was to consider the following assumption: *Therapists can't change clients, clients can only change themselves.* How might that be helpful? The therapist answered that it made him think more about what was going on with John, particularly about the death of John's mother. This therapist's message at the end of the first session is evidence that he was aware that John was in the midst of intense mourning for his mother. However, he believed that he should not talk about it with the client because, first, it would distract from talking about positives and the future; second, it dealt with John's emotions; and third, it had not been identified as a problem or a goal. When the therapist was encouraged to address the mourning it proved to be the key to the solution. John started to cry and to vent about how much he missed his mother. He spoke about how he never realized how much his mother had compensated for his father's personality, and how he had no idea how he would manage without her in the future. This outpouring of emotion prompted the therapist to put aside thoughts about intervention at the time and just to be supportive. Toward the end of the session John made a confession. He told the therapist that he felt more stressed from guilt than from anger at his father because he had been wishing all along that his father had died instead of his mother.

Notice how the therapist's shift from a formulaic concept of SFT to one driven by emotion and theory lead to a more trusting relationship in which John felt safe to confess his shameful feelings. When these feelings were not judged but understood and normalized, John expressed some relief. The therapist then wondered how John thought his guilt was affecting his tolerance of his father's behavior. John made the connection that the more hostile his father was, the more guilt he felt, and the more guilt he felt the less he could tolerate his father's hostility.

John's new understanding led to a redefinition of what he wanted from therapy. He now declared he would feel comfortable if he could reduce his guilt about his shameful feelings from the present level of 10 to below 5. Once John was clear about that he began to find behaviors that helped him. He talked to his wife about his feelings and discovered that she and their children had had similar thoughts. John also began attending church more regularly. He confessed to his pastor, who responded in a comforting rather than judgmental manner. As John's guilt decreased, his grief increased, resulting in a gradual acceptance of his loss. This made room for some empathy for his father and a new connection with him around loving memories about his mother. At the end of treatment, 6 months later, John reported that to his surprise his father was showing some signs of becoming softer. "From a position of true respect, techniques per se become superfluous, as action appropriate to this situation is generated from the simple act of paying attention to what is needed" (Simon, 1996, p. 53).

All good therapy takes place in the context of a trusting relationship. The specific manner in which the therapist guides that relationship is determined by his or her theoretical orientation. Thus a psychodynamic therapist, who is guided by assumptions that clients must develop insight to change, will make different choices in conversation with clients than will a behavioral therapist, who believes that behavior changes as a result of new learning, or reconditioning. If solution-focused therapists assume change occurs through language, and that is understood to mean no more than asking certain questions, disappointing results are probable (Fraser, 1995).

BEYOND TECHNIQUE TO THEORY

The suggestion that the road to the more successful use of a minimalist model is to complicate it with theory will undoubtedly seem paradoxical to some readers. Many clinicians, eager to improve their clinical skills, look for more ideas about "how" to talk to clients not "why." Workshop participants are eager for videotapes or live demonstrations of how the presenter works and may quickly become restless and bored with theoretical explanations. Theory is an abstraction that appears, at times, to be far removed from the actual conversations we have with clients. However, it is the only solution to a problem many therapists struggle with but are reluctant to admit that they have, namely, that they often sit in a session and do not know what to do next.

Theory becomes less formidable when we realize that it is part of everything we do well in life. Driving a car safely requires some theory that goes beyond obeying traffic signals. Playing tennis, golf, sailing, and other sports entail theoretical assumptions about our bodies and the physical properties of the air around us. Good cooking is more than following a recipe. It requires assumptions about what will happen to certain foods when they are subjected to heat, or when they are mixed with each other. Of course, people can do all these activities without understanding the underlying theory, but it is less likely that they will excel at what they do or transcend technical skills to become artists. Because therapy is a professional endeavor that brings with it a huge responsibility toward other human beings it is worthy of our best efforts.

This book proposes a theory and basic assumptions for SFT that refutes the frequent accusation that SFT is formulaic and mechanical. It diverts emphasis from techniques to the therapist–client relationship, so important for successful outcome (Bachelor & Horvath, 1999; Beyebach, Morejon, Palenzuela, & Rodriguez-Arias, 1996; Hubble, Duncan, & Miller, 1999) and to the use of emotions. Less attention to techniques helps therapists avoid two common pitfalls: withdrawing attention from clients to ruminate about what question to ask or asking the questions at inappropriate times.

A BRIEF HISTORICAL DETOUR

SFT was originally conceived as Brief Family Therapy in Milwaukee, Wisconsin, in the late 1970s (de Shazer, 1982). As such, it can be thought of as a younger sibling of the brief therapy model developed at the Mental Research Institute in Palo Alto, California (Fisch, Weakland, & Segal, 1982; Ray, 2000; Watzlawick & Weakland, 1977; Watzlawick, Weakland, & Fisch, 1974). The Mental Research Institute model has roots in the work on paradox and human communication led by Gregory Bateson (Bateson, Jackson, Haley, & Weakland, 1956; Jackson, 1959) and Milton Erickson's ideas about circumventing resistance in hypnotherapy (Erickson, 1977; Erickson & Rossi, 1979). However, while the Mental Research Institute's interventions were targeted at interrupting interactional patterns therapists identified as faulty attempts at solution, the Brief Family Therapy Center's ecosystemic approach (de Shazer, 1982; Keeney, 1979) was more collaborative, and based on the assumption that "the family has the solution" (Norum, 2000). Therapists together with clients were considered a therapeutic suprasystem that generated new, nonproblematic interactional patterns for the family system. This mind-set was more in the tradition of the postmodern era that followed, in which constructivism and social constructionism[1] became dominant influences in the field of family therapy.

The shift from problem-focused Brief Family Therapy to SFT occurred in 1982, in a random manner. As I remember the incident, there

---

1. "Constructivism" is defined here as "a relativistic point of view that emphasizes the subjective construction of reality. [It] implies that what we see in families may be based as much on our preconditions as on what's actually going on" (Nichols & Schwartz, 1995, p. 590). It is represented by theorists such as Paul Watzlawick (1984), Humberto Maturana (1980), Heinz von Foerster (1981), and Ernst von Glasserfeld (1984). Each person constructs his or her own image of what reality is through language (Anderson, 1997). "Social constructionism" (Gergen, 1982, 1991, 1994), with which constructivism is confused, goes a step beyond this to assert that individual constructs are shaped entirely through conversations with others.

were a number of core group members behind the mirror formulating an intervention message for a family that had come with their rebellious teenage daughter and was not reporting any progress by the end of the second or third session. The father and mother were only interested in reporting all the things their daughter continued to do wrong and diverted from any questions about exceptions. The daughter remained sullen. That day, one of us behind the mirror—and there are strong opinions about who it actually was—said, "Why don't we ask them to make a list of what they *don't* want to change for next time?" We all agreed, and were pleasantly surprised when the parents and the daughter came back with sizable lists of what they appreciated about each other. What was more surprising, however, were the positive changes all three family members reported. They all agreed that there had been less tension in the home. The parents felt their daughter's attitude had changed for the better and the daughter felt that her parents had stopped being so critical. After assigning this task to the next few clients at the end of the first session and getting similar results, a research study was designed (de Shazer, 1985, p. 147). The results indicated that the concrete changes clients reported in the second session generally had little to do with their description of the problem or complaints in the first session. Moreover, these changes could often be amplified to become solutions. This discovery shifted our attention to the interview as a locus of intervention (Lipchik, 1988a, 1988b; Lipchik & de Shazer, 1986; Penn, 1982, 1985; Tomm, 1987a, 1987b). The message and task at the end of the session now reinforced the process that was generated during the interview. Gradually, these future-oriented, solution-focused questions overshadowed all else that was essential for conducting good therapy, particularly the emphasis on cooperating with how clients cooperate, which is defined as follows: "each family (individual or couple) shows a unique way of attempting to cooperate, and the therapist's job becomes first to describe that particular manner to himself that the family shows, and then, to cooperate with the family's way" (de Shazer, 1982, pp. 9–10).

In an effort to conserve this relational/interactional context for the techniques in a theoretically sound manner (Lipchik, 1993), I revisited the interpersonal theory of psychiatrist Harry Stack Sullivan (Chapman, 1973; Sullivan, 1953c, 1953d). Sullivan's thinking fit the constructivist frame (Cushman, 1995) because it denied objective reality in therapy, except for what can be "directly observed (in the present) in the context of interpersonal relationships [the therapeutic relationship]" (Chapman, 1973, p. 70). Consequently, Sullivan defined the therapist's role as that of a "participating observer" (1953d, p. 18) whose job was to engage with patients in a process toward more functional interpersonal behaviors rather than to sit silently and interpret. Diagnostic labels also did not fit Sullivan's thinking. Problems and solutions were no more or less than an individual's degree of emotional discomfort ("anxiety") or comfort ("security") in interpersonal relationships. Like Maturana and Varela (1987) much later, Sullivan (1953d) considered these human relationships from a biological perspective, an interdependence of living organisms with their environment.

In 1984, the Brief Family Therapy Center engaged in a project in artificial intelligence—"BRIEFER"— to develop an "expert system," a computer program to assist in formulating a task in the first session (Goodman, 1986; Goodman, Gingerich, & de Shazer, 1989). For that purpose, we engaged in a step-by-step analysis of how we made decisions in relation to clients, both as the interviewer and team member behind the mirror. This exercise really illuminated the importance of nonverbal language and emotions as a context for, and connection between, questions and answers. Yet it stimulated the development of a theory of solution (de Shazer, 1988) that was essentially a decision tree for the solution-focused therapeutic process. In retrospect, this further depersonalization of SFT spurred me on to counter this trend (Lipchik, 1993, 1994, 1997, 1999; Lipchik & Kubicki, 1996). My search for a theoretically sound way to do so continued after I left the Brief Family Therapy Center in 1988 and started ICF Consultants, Inc., with Marilyn Bonjean, in Milwaukee.

The theory of cognition developed by the Chilean biologists Humberto Maturana and Francisco Varela (1980, 1987; Varela, 1989) that stimulated the field of family therapy in the early 1980s (Dell, 1982, 1985; Efran & Lukens, 1985; Efran, Lukens, & Lukens, 1990; Ludewig, 1992; Parry, 1984; Simon, 1985) eventually provided the basis of a suitable framework. Maturana himself has describes this theory as a "metatheory," which provides a way of unifying all the disparate theoretical schools of family therapy (Simon, 1985, p. 4).

In studies of the retina of frogs conducted in the 1950s, Humberto Maturana discovered that the image a frog's brain received when visualizing a fly is the result of the structure of its eye, not an objective representation of the fly in the world outside. This discovery had a considerable impact on the understanding of perception and eventually led to a theory of cognition (1980, 1987) that suggests that our reality, or what we know, depends on who we are in terms of our structure, as well as our interactions with others.

Maturana and Varela's theory describes living systems as "auto-poietic," organized to survive and re-create themselves. This survival and re-creation depends on structure coupling, a state of interdependence with the environment and/or other living systems. Mutual survival is constantly challenged by internal perturbations as well as mutual external perturbations and depends on mutual adaptation. Perturbations cannot change another living system; they can only trigger the possibility of change. That change depends on the particular organization of the system (structure determinism). Thus, if two or more interdependent systems cannot conserve their basic survival needs in interaction with each other, their relationship will end. For example, if the heart fails it will destroy the respiratory system, the vascular system, and the renal system and a person will die.

According to this theory, the development of language occurred late in the evolution of living systems and distinguishes humans from other living mechanisms. Language is seen as part of a person's individual structure but a mutually dependent action, "a phenomenon that takes place in the recursion of linguistic interactions—linguistic coordinations of linguistic coordinations of action" (Maturana & Varela, 1987, p. 211). In other words, each human being has a closed neural network that generates its own information (Efran et al., 1990, p. 67), but language is an act of mutual adaptation, or consensus about meaning between people and social groups.

If I go to a restaurant and order a sandwich on toasted bread, I already have information in my system about what toasted bread means from previous linguistic interactions. I may have learned what "bread" and "toast" means from my mother when I was a little child. If the waiter in the present situation does not understand what toasted bread means we have to act to coordinate the meaning. Another way of saying it is that we have to adapt to each other in a way that our relationship can survive: that the waiter can fill my order in a manner that will satisfy me, and thereby fulfill his job in a way that will not get him fired. The coordination of the meaning of toasted bread depends on whether we both speak the same language. If we do not, can we understand each other in some other way, perhaps with gestures or nonverbal cues? If we both speak the same language but the waiter is not familiar with toasted bread, will I be able to explain it, and will he have the capacity to understand my explanation so we can maintain a mutually beneficial connection?

There were two aspects of Maturana and Varela's work that were particularly attractive to me as a solution-focused therapist. One was the idea that survival and adaptation is an interdependent process between living systems that is based on conserving what these interdependent living systems need individually to survive; in other words, it is essential to build on what is working. The other was that we cannot know or act without biological dynamics we call emotions. In particular, the emotion Maturana and Varela (1987) call "love," or the acceptance of another beside us in our daily living, is considered the biological basis for social life that allows for the continuation of relationships and of life itself. This strength-based idea is strikingly similar to Harry Stack Sullivan's concept of "consensual validation" whereby people "attend to one another's emotional states and exchange coded information regarding what is proper and improper, anxiety provoking or soothing" (Cushman, 1995, p. 178).

A SOLUTION-FOCUSED THEORY

What follows is a theory that grew out of my personal experience of what works in SFT. I think of it as a constructivist theory that conserves some interactional/strategic concepts and integrates them with a biological perspective that includes emotions.

> *Human beings are unique in their genetic heritage and social development. Their capacity to change is determined by these factors and their interactions with others. Problems are present life situations experienced as emotional discomfort with self, and in relation to others. Change occurs through language when recognition of exceptions and existing and potential strengths create new actions.*

The assumptions made from this statement shape the therapist's attitude toward clients and guide the therapist–client relationship. Notice that these assumptions often overlap, or flow into each other even though they address different points. Thus, they have a way of reinforcing each other.

SOLUTION-FOCUSED ASSUMPTIONS

1. *Every client is unique.* This relates to the theory that living systems (clients) are structure determined. When solution-focused thera-

pists keep this in mind, it helps them resist the natural temptation to think that they know what the solution should be for a particular client's problem because it worked in a similar case, or because it works for them in their personal life. Because every client is unique, every relationship is unique. One couple's relationship problems after the birth of their first child may be solved when the wife allows the husband to participate more in child care while another's solution may be that the husband and wife each has an evening out once a week.

SFT is a constructivist model. Considering the use of the same intervention is a linear way of thinking that implies causality and focuses on content rather than process. The best way to ensure the probability of the fastest and most fitting solution for clients is to treat them as unique and to remain "curious" (Cecchin, 1987).

Of course, this is not meant to imply that personal or professional experience does not have a place in therapy. However, it should only be applied after we have tried everything we know to help the client access his or her own information, and then in a tentative manner, like "Some people find that it is helpful to . . . " or "If you were to consider . . ., do you think that could be helpful?"

2. *Clients have the inherent strength and resources to help themselves.* This assumption represents the heart of the solution-focused philosophy and is perhaps one of the most difficult ones for therapists to remember. As members of the helping profession we consider it our responsibility to relieve our clients' pain as quickly as possible. We become not unlike protective parents who guide too much in an effort to prevent their children from getting hurt instead of helping them to use their own resources to take care of themselves. Such parenting does not empower and build confidence!

Maturana's answer to the question "What is the purpose of therapy?" offers a helpful perspective to support this assumption. With regard to structure coupling, he said that therapy should generate dynamics of interaction in which people recover something in themselves (self-respect, love, legitimacy) as well as in others (1996). Considered from the position of therapists, it suggests we look for and emphasize our resources of acceptance, empathy, and respect for clients.

From a more practical point of view, this assumption is a reminder that the simple act of being alive and finding their way to our office represents clients' strengths. They have survived physically and emotionally so far, and we must now join them in continuing their life to the best of their ability. However, the story of that survival can often be so fraught with difficulties and pain that it can make us feel devastated and hopeless. At those times, thoughts of "This is horrendous," "I can't be helpful here," or "I wouldn't know where to begin," are best counteracted with the assumption that clients have the strengths and resources to help themselves. This thinking then automatically leads to a response such as, "You really have a lot to deal with right now. How have you been coping with all this?" This response focuses on resources immediately as well as benefiting the therapist–client relationship with its message of understanding and positive regard.

3. *Nothing is all negative.* This assumption is supported by Maturana and Varela's idea that there can be no change without conservation. Our clients usually perceive their situation as all bad, and they are not aware of exceptions and their own resources. They say things such as "I must get rid of my anxiety" not realizing that some anxiety is an asset in many situations. As therapists we, too, are not immune to this either–or thinking at times. Thus, when clients present us with situations that involve personal losses, poor health, financial struggles, and legal problems all at once, which they sometimes do, this assumption directs us toward thinking, "Yes, but what has kept them going and how can we preserve that and build on it?" This thinking directs us toward coping questions, which are much more empathic and sensitive in extreme situations than to ask, "What's still OK in your life?" when nothing seems to be.

4. *There is no such thing as resistance.* "Resistant" is what therapists call clients who do not accept the therapist's point of view about how they should change. The whole concept of therapists labeling clients' behavior does not fit with SFT or postmodern thinking in general. A client cannot be resistant; the therapist simply does not understand how to trigger (perturbate) change in a way that allows the client to respond adaptively. Therefore, the therapist must continue to look to the client for better understanding of what will work for him or her.

Maturana uses the term "orthogonal interaction" to describe the therapeutic process. It means relating to a person in such a way that he or she must generate a new or infrequently used response. The interaction perturbates in a way that forces new patterns to emerge (Efran & Blumberg, 1994).

However, though resistance is not a fitting solution-focused concept, the word "resistance" is still a good description of what solution-focused therapists often feel in interaction with clients. What therapist is not familiar with the experience of feeling his or her body tense as a client replies with "yes, but!" to everything that is discussed? We notice that we are not sitting back in our usual relaxed position but leaning toward the client stiffly. Our voice may be louder than usual and our throat may feel tight. We feel as if we are working too hard. If we can call on this assumption at such a moment it will help us sit back in our chair, take a slow breath, and turn to the client and ask, "What do you think would be best for you at this time so things can get better?" This is helpful for us, as well as for the client, because of the positive effect it will have on the emotional climate.

5. *You cannot change clients; they can only change themselves.* Once in a rare while, every solution-focused therapist experiences the feeling of being in a power struggle with a client, or of trying too hard to get an idea across. The belief that living systems are "informationally closed" and cannot be changed from the outside supports this assumption that prevents, or corrects, such lapses.

An example that comes to mind is a situation in which a mother, whose son was placed in residential treatment after sexually abusing a younger sibling, was ordered to work with a family therapist toward reunification. The boy was making excellent progress and the agency purchasing the services was anxious to have the boy discharged from the expensive residential treatment. However, in spite of solution-focused techniques the family therapist could not get the mother to stand behind her stated intentions to make the necessary changes in the home, and herself, so the home would be pronounced safe for the younger sibling. Colleagues he consulted urged the therapist to stop being "solution focused" and to intensify the mother's anxiety about losing her son to get her to change. Instead, this therapist chose to look back to some solution-focused literature from the late 1980s, and ran across this assumption. As a result, he decided he would change himself to make a difference. He decided to assume responsibility by apologizing to the mother for not having been helpful enough for her to meet other people's expectations for her and asked her to help him understand more about how he could do that. In response, the mother became very emotional and expressed some ambivalence about reunification. She confessed guilt about not wanting to make efforts to make changes that she believed had little chance of working. This confession opened up the opportunity for the therapist to help her deal with her guilt and work on some other options for the future that offered more hope. The boy was placed in foster care while the family continued to work toward reunification. An environment that indicated support, rather than blame, gradually led to changes that allowed for reunification.

When clients seem stuck it is often helpful to convey to them that we understand their feelings. Maturana cautions against trying to change clients by means of logic without a mutual agreement about the underlying emotions because of his belief that preferences (emotions) determine actions (Maturana, 1988, p. 17).

6. *SFT goes slowly.* SFT is a brief model, similar to the one developed at the Mental Research Institute Brief Therapy Clinic. I have dropped the word "brief" deliberately to dispel false assumptions. The foregoing assumption was originally developed to counteract the belief that "brief" implies "quickly." Brief therapy models can usually provide effective, long-lasting treatment in shorter periods than other therapy models. However, the brevity will be the result of the best-fitting intervention for a particular client, not speedy application of technique. Premature use of technique can prolong treatment because it may focus on complaints that are not related to what the client really wants from therapy.

SFT is also used slowly for cases that require therapeutic support for years. Episodes of intense contact during crisis interspersed with mild ongoing support can yield surprising improvement in functioning over time if the focus remains on small goals identified by clients and worked on in a secure emotional climate.

This assumption is primarily a reminder to us to be patient with ourselves. We are doing SFT even if we are just tending to the environment clients need in order to change.

7. *There is no cause and effect.* The concept of cause and effect does not exist in a constructivist world because it implies the existence of some objective truth. Instead, problems and solutions are viewed as the unpredictable events of living. Thus, we must not allow ourselves to be seduced by clients to join them in thinking "why does this problem exist?" but direct our efforts toward "What has to be different in the future?" On the other hand, we must be prepared to join our clients in talking about cause and effect if that is the only way they can think about solution.

For example, a client reports that a self-help book she read last week is responsible for her suddenly feeling like her old self again after several months of feeling depressed. The therapist's experience has been that she has reported gradual signs of improvement but has been reluctant to admit to them. What is important here is that the client found a way to change. If the client prefers to believe the cause of her change is a book rather than therapy, that cause-and-effect thinking is the client's way of changing and needs to be accepted. For this client, change in the context of a relationship with a therapist was not an option at that time.

There are some strong beliefs in the mental health field that the experience of sexual and physical abuse are directly responsible for emotional problems in later life. Undoubtedly, such terrible events have an impact on the victim's life; however, it is impossible to determine a direct link because one can always find clients who exhibit similar symptoms without having been abused. As long as mental health professionals do not have diagnostic tools like physicians, such as imaging techniques and blood analyses, cause-and-effect thinking is a road no solution-focused therapist should travel.

When clients search for causes it is useful to ask them how knowing the cause will be helpful for them in solving their problem. They usually say it will help them understand. The question, "If you could solve your problem without understanding, would that be all right?" usually offers another perspective that many clients have never considered.

8. *Solutions do not necessarily have anything to do with the problem.* This assumption was developed at Brief Family Therapy Center in 1982, as a result of the shift from problem to solution focus, described earlier. At the time, it was discovered that the question "What don't you want to change about the situation that you came about" generated positive differences outside the problem description. It seemed to trigger creative actions in clients who were unable to change when they thought about what they wanted to change.

Again, we are reminded not to think cause and effect. In life, like in therapy, change is inevitable as well as unpredictable. For example, a man or woman who is bored on the job may become increasingly lethargic and ineffective. An unexpected stimulus outside work, such as a hobby, sport, or new relationship, may result in a general change of attitude that affects his or her perception of and performance on the job as well. Searching for solutions only in relation to the problem can seriously constrain progress.

9. *Emotions are part of every problem and every solution.* For theoretical and practical reasons the Mental Research Institute and solution-focused model have had a cognitive-behavioral focus and eschewed talk about feelings except for joining. However, if language is thought of as an action from which emotion is inseparable, then clients emotions are as much a subject of therapy than their thoughts and behaviors. Given that theory, the failure to talk to clients about their feelings, and to connect with them on that level, could limit our understanding of them, their understanding of themselves, and the possibilities for solutions.

This assumption reminds us that emotions are part of language and are essential for our clients' process of decision making (Damasio, 1994; Maturana & Varela, 1987). This assumption also reminds us to be attentive to the emotional climate in which our relationship with clients takes place (see Chapter 2, this volume), first, because security, rather than anxiety, is the emotional state people seek (Sullivan, 1953d) and are most relaxed in, and second, because a state of relaxation makes people more open to their own resources and new information (Erickson, 1977).

If a client describes being stuck with his doctoral dissertation in engineering in terms of time, space, family obligations, and computer problems, the best way to cooperate with him would probably be to use language and concepts that fit his concrete world view. However, if that does not make a difference for him, introducing talk about his emotional state given the problem would be productive.

We connect with people emotionally in a nonverbal way as well, and some clients may be aware of their emotions but are more comfortable not talking about them. As therapists, it is our responsibility to be sensitive to our clients' comfort levels and to respect them. However, the important point is to convey that we understand what they are telling us in as much depth as possible.

10. *Change is constant and inevitable; a small change can lead to bigger changes.* The Mental Research Institute and SFT have always viewed problems as the inevitable ups and down of living. Some people overcome their problems by going to therapy and others recover spontaneously (Bergin & Lambert, 1978). Forty percent of clients are believed to recover because of extratherapeutic factors (Lambert, 1992). We really have no proof that those who seek help would not have improved without that help.

Our lives are subject to constant change given our complex network of relationships ranging from our nuclear family to people across the globe and circumstances such as wars, weather, and astrophysical phenomena, many of which are beyond our control or unknown. Change in any of them has the potential of affecting our lives.

An awareness of this certainty about uncertainty, combined with the belief in clients' inherent resources, helps the solution-focused therapist maintain a hopeful attitude regardless of the difficulties clients relate. Thus, when we feel overwhelmed by a client's story and feel as stuck as the client about what to do, the first step is to realize change is inevitable; the second step is to engage with the client about doing something, no matter how small, that the client thinks will make a difference. In a situation that appears hopeless or overwhelming, a small step can provide a sense of control that has been missing. Taking action, no matter how minor, can feel like movement out of total stuckness, and therefore it generates hope. It is up to us not to be too ambitious about our clients' small steps, and to keep the clients from being too ambitious, because something as seemingly insignificant as combing one's hair differently, making a phone call to an old friend, or eating a meal with someone rather than alone can lead to bigger changes.

All of us have had the experience of being overwhelmed with so much work that it seems too much to tackle. The best solution is usually to make a list, prioritize, and beginning working. Suddenly the entire workload seems manageable. A small change can lead to bigger change!

11. *One can't change the past so one should concentrate on the future.* This assumption is so self-evident and yet not easy to remember at all times. Accepting the assumption that language is an action in the present supports the belief that change can also happen only in the present.

Clients often say they will know they do not have to come to therapy anymore when they understand their past actions that resulted in the problem. They seem to believe that insight is necessary for a solution. Some clients even persist in trying to understand "why" after they have reached their goal.

A common occurrence in couple therapy is that even though both partners want to stay together they are held back from progress because one or both keep harping on hurtful events from the past. Solution-focused therapists must avoid getting caught in that futile process and find ways to help clients forgive, if not forget, for the sake of their future.

Another no-win process that frequently occurs in therapy is that clients obsess about the wrongs they perceive their parents to have perpetrated against them when they were children. Not only can these wrongs not be changed, but they may be memories of childhood perceptions that might have been experienced differently at another stage of life.

A useful way of working with clients who persist in harping on the past is to say "I realize that it is difficult for you to forget (or forgive) the past (pain, disappointment, etc.), but what do you think you would need now, or in the future, to come to terms with the fact that it happened, or to begin to put it behind you?"

Assumptions shape our attitudes toward clients and therefore our relationship with them. They help us make decisions about what to do. The assumption that clients have strengths will make us ask questions about them. The assumption that all problems and solutions involve emotions will remind us to be empathic and encouraging. When a client reports a relapse after several good weeks we may be tempted to join him or her in searching for reasons why this happened. Instead these solution-focused assumptions provide a source for shaping a positive attitude in us, and our clients, by prompting us to ask: "Since you first described the problem you came in about you have made some progress. This cannot not have had some effect on the present situation. What is different about the situation now than when you first came in?" These connections between theory, assumptions, and practice will be pointed out throughout this book.

CONCLUSION

As SFT has become increasingly atheoretical the skepticism, particularly about how it is practiced, has grown (Efron & Veenendaal, 1993; Kleckner, Frank, Bland, Amendt, & Bryant, 1992; Lipchik, 1994; S. D. Miller, 1994; Nylund & Corsiglia, 1994). The theory described in this chapter was developed to provide an alternative way of conceptualizing and practicing SFT, one that leaves less questions about its legitimacy and worth (Cecchin, Lane, & Ray, 1994). In keeping with the idea that change must involve conservation, this version of SFT reintroduces past aspects of SFT and integrates them with formerly unrelated ones. The biological component paves the way for integrating future findings from neuroscience and other medical areas that can help us help our clients more effectively.

I have based my reasoning about misconceptions about SFT on the-oretical changes, but I want to emphasize that managed care companies should not be relieved of some blame too (Hoyt & Friedman, 1998). The endorsement by managed care companies of SFT as the brief treat-ment of choice resulted in a plethora of 1- and 2-day workshops de-signed to give the participants something useful to take back to their practice. In such circumstances, techniques take precedence and theoreti-cal context only complicates matters. As these trainings proliferated, their main sound bytes have come to define SFT.

As therapists we should not expect our work to be a smooth ride. Therefore, we must keep searching for ways to cushion that ride for our clients and ourselves.

2

The Therapist–Client Relationship

About 10 years ago, my business partner Marilyn Bonjean and I became increasingly interested in learning more about what is most helpful to our clients. We decided to conduct an informal study for that purpose and developed a short questionnaire that was given to clients at the beginning of their second session and at every session thereafter. The questionnaire asked clients to evaluate if they were better, the same, or worse since the last session, and whether their experience was the result of anything that had occurred in their last session. They were asked to briefly describe anything they believed to have influenced any changes. The therapists answered a parallel questionnaire at the end of every session, starting with the first session. They had to predict whether the clients would report being better, the same, or worse, and to briefly describe why. We gathered material for about a year. We did not look at the completed questionnaires until a case was closed.

The results surprised us. Clients' reports suggested that they valued the content of sessions far less than the process. Without exception they associated their progress with feeling understood, supported, accepted, and listened to. Therapists, on the other hand, predicted changes based on what had been discussed in sessions, what clients said was new or different, or on homework assignments. Our outcome evaluation was consistent with the results obtained in studies conducted for SFT (Beyebach et al., 2000; DeJong & Hopwood, 1996; Gingerich & Eisengart, 2000; Kiser, 1988; Kiser & Nunnally, 1990; McKeel, 1996; Metcalf, Thomas, Duncan, Miller, & Hubble, 1996) that found that about 80% of clients said they made significant improvement during therapy.

This chapter describes how to establish and maintain a relationship with clients that makes them feel supported while they adapt or change. This process is examined from the perspective of the client as well as the therapist.

RESEARCH FINDINGS

The informal study conducted at our clinic is in line with current thinking about the importance of the therapist–client relationship for therapy (Beyebach et al., 1996; Horvath & Symonds, 1991; Hubble et al., 1999; Orlinsky, Grawe, & Parks, 1994; Patterson, 1984; Turnell & Lipchik, 1999). Hubble and colleagues (1996) cite Lambert (1992) as estimating that the major determinants of outcome in therapy (40%) are extra-therapeutic factors, that is, internal and external factors clients bring to therapy; 30% of outcome is determined by factors related to the therapist–client relationship, such as caring, acceptance, encouragement, while only 15% is determined by factors particular to the therapeutic model and techniques; the other 15% consist of placebo effect.

THE SOLUTION-FOCUSED
THERAPIST–CLIENT RELATIONSHIP

In the context of the theory presented in Chapter 1, the therapist–client relationship represents a structure coupling between two unique human beings cast in complementary roles, the professional helper and the client who is experiencing him- or herself as unable to resolve a problem. The different knowledge and expectations that each contributes constitutes the relationship at any moment in time. However, it is the responsibility of the therapist to use his or her theoretical assumptions to guide that relationship for the client's benefit.

I think of the solution-focused therapist–client relationship like a mutual journey to the client's solution. The client takes the lead in deciding where to go. The client contributes how he or she cooperates, his or her readiness for change, and his or her expectations. The therapist acts as a guide with questions and answers carefully chosen to help the client clarify his or her direction or change it for one that is more likely to lead to his or her destination.

The underpinning for therapist–client relationships, regardless of orientation, is trust. Clients must trust that we are committed to helping them without hurting them. Given the strength-based philosophy of SFT, that means getting clients to trust us to help them trust themselves. This is a delicate balancing act that requires us to gauge when to intervene and when not to. A long time ago (Lipchik & Vega, 1984), I likened the process to teaching someone to ride a bicycle. You provide security by running closely behind the person as he or she tries to keep from falling. However, you have to choose carefully when to let the person rely on his or her own sense of balance and when to steady the person by holding the back of the seat.

THE EMOTIONAL CLIMATE

Ideally, the therapist–client relationship should create an emotional climate in which therapy can take place as smoothly as possible. Most clients describe their problems in predominantly feeling-related words and actions. Therefore, the first step a solution-focused therapist can take to connect on the emotional level is to assume a relaxed, friendly stance, much as one would with a guest in one's own home. Questions about traffic problems on the way to the office, difficulties locating the office, and the effects of the weather are always useful. Next, clients should be invited to talk about their feelings about therapy before further inquiries into demographics or history. For example, "Is this your first experience with therapy?" If so, "That can be uncomfortable for some people." "Is there anything you would like to know about what we will be doing?" If the client is visible anxious, "It is hard to come to a stranger to talk about things that trouble you. Is there anything I could do to make you feel more comfortable?"

I routinely ask clients what they would like to know about me and the agency before I start asking for information about them. This is usually met with pleasant surprise, and some clients take advantage of this question and others do not. These steps begin to define a relationship of acceptance, understanding, and mutual respect that is emotionally comfortable. As Erickson has taught us so masterfully, it is natural to relax in the presence of someone who does not challenge us.

Figures 1 and 2 portray the therapist–client interactions that generate the emotional climate. Both diagrams should be understood to represent a process that begins the moment therapists and clients meet and lasts for the duration of the relationship. The emotional climate, once it appears to provide safety and comfort for the client, cannot be assumed to remain stable throughout treatment. It must be monitored at all times and maintained lest it disturb progress.

THE CLIENT'S POSITION

Clients enter the therapeutic relationship feeling vulnerable and helpless. They are not yet aware that their memories, perceptions, fears, and expectations are valuable resources and hold the key to their solution. The degree to which they can access and/or use this information to clarify what they need and want affects progress. The case of John, at the beginning of Chapter 1, is an example. When John felt safe enough to talk about his guilt with the therapist it opened the way to a revised goal and self-initiated steps toward the solution.

Most clients who come to therapy feel a lack of control over their life. They are caught in a downward spiral of hopelessness. As indicated in Figure 1 they fear judgment and the unknown and guard themselves in relation to the therapist. They are focused on the problem, what they, or others, have done wrong in the past, and perceive their situation as "all bad" or "all good."

Clients often feel uncertain about how to conduct themselves when they first enter therapy. Some expect the therapist will "do something to make them change." These doubts can feel threatening, even for those who desire change. Change also implies existing inadequacies that one may want to avoid admitting or exposing. As therapists, we must convey the understanding that change, or the potential for it, may evoke some anxiety and watch for signs of it throughout therapy. When we find evidence of such anxiety the solution-focused manner of helping is to normalize it and help clients accept, rather than fight, the feelings. For example, "It is normal that you feel (confused, uncertain, uncomfortable, anxious). It may actually serve a good purpose because it is telling you to slow down and give yourself some time to get used to the changes that are possible (or that have occurred) and to think carefully about how you want to move on. It is always best to go slowly."

THE THERAPIST'S POSITION

In contrast to the client's hopeless and fearful position, the solution-focused therapist, who has expertise the client does not have, must be careful not to control, influence, and advise. The best position to assume is

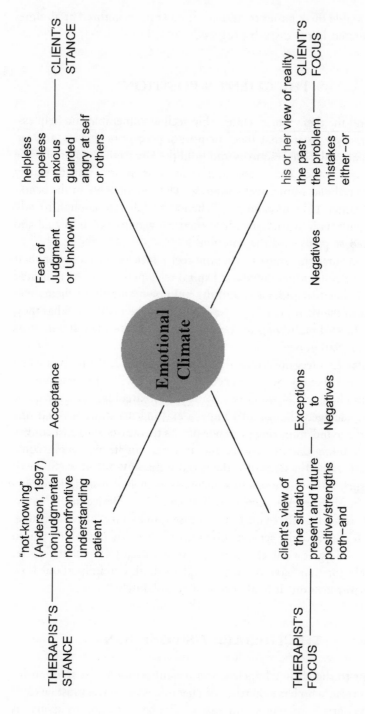

FIGURE 1. Therapist–client interaction.

one of "not knowing" (Anderson, 1997). This is a stance of "humility about what one knows. In effect, [one in which] a therapist is more interested in learning what a client has to say than in pursuing, telling, validating, or promoting his or her knowledge or preoccupations" (Anderson, 1997, p. 136). There should be no reluctance to ask for clarification to the point of sounding obtuse. Differences in what clients mean may be minute, but they are important for focusing on what clients really want. Timing is also of the essence. Interrupting clients to ask a question, or introduce a new idea, must be done carefully lest it feels disrespectful or rejecting.

The solution-focused position of acceptance, conveyed through an understanding, nonjudgmental, and nonconfrontational stance, should not be misinterpreted to mean that we never contest what clients say. Most of the times the solution-focused therapist can start therapy by just listening in an accepting manner and gradually focusing on what clients say they want. Sometimes, however, clients tell us things about their lives that we have a professional obligation to address regardless of our theoretical stance, such as child abuse or homicidal or suicidal thoughts. These issues can be addressed in a manner befitting solution-focused philosophy and with an eye to protecting the emotional climate. An example might be the disclosure of physical abuse:

> "I know how hard you try to be a good parent and to teach your daughter to behave, and how frustrated you must be that she doesn't listen, but I wonder whether you know that hitting her with a belt is against the law. It is something I am obligated to report to Child Protective Services unless you report it yourself. If you do that on your own, it will be seen as a sign that you are taking responsibility and that you want to change. That will be helpful to you in their decision about how to handle your situation and I will do all I can to work with you on other ways to make her behave."

Generally, the therapist–client relationship is less jeopardized when clients report to authorities rather than the therapist.

Later in the course of therapy, when more trust has been established, there is generally less danger of harming the emotional climate. Nevertheless, we must never relax our attention to what appears to be going on with clients so that we can respond in a manner that will maintain a positive emotional climate. When we notice clients missing appointments or appearing less relaxed in sessions, it is best to ask whether there is anything *we* can do to help correct that rather than blaming the client. A client may confess that she is disappointed that there is not more change, or that the conversations do not deal with what she really wants to talk about. This response calls for an apology and an inquiry about the client's view of what would correct the situation. This interchange can be a valuable lesson about assertiveness for clients as well as moving therapy forward.

Conversations between clients and therapists have the potential of yielding much more information for solutions in a favorable emotional climate. Clients are usually careful about what they reveal at first. The less defensive they become the more information becomes available. Figure 2 illustrates the therapist–client exchange during a single session as well as the whole course of therapy. The therapist asks a question that generates a response of old or new information for the client and the therapist, as well as directing the therapist toward the next question to be asked. In this recursive pattern the therapist must choose whether to reflect, nod, ask for clarification, or use a technique, based on his or her judgment of whether it will keep the client emotionally comfortable.

For example, Tamara comes in to make a decision whether to leave her husband or not. He is not interested in couple counseling. Among the complaints of insensitivity, laziness, and irresponsibility was one that he spends their limited joint income without consulting her. The therapist asked, "What do you do when your husband goes out to buy a new electronic toy without telling you first?" Tamara answers, "I get very upset." The therapist accepts this with a nod but wants more information. She asks "What is it like when you get upset?" Tamara answers that she gets really disappointed, and sometimes she cries and asks why he is doing this. The therapist now has information that suggests the client's reaction is a fairly normal one under the circumstances.

In the next session the therapist and Tamara continue to talk about the present and future pros and cons of Tamara's relationship with her husband to facilitate her decision. The therapist continues to be accepting of Tamara's version of her responses to her husband's behavior. Toward the end of the third session, Tamara reports another one of her husband's compulsive spending incidents and the therapist responds with, "This must be so hard for you!" Tamara answers, "It is, but I wish I would not lose it so badly." The therapist is surprised by this statement. "What do you mean by not losing it so badly?" she asks. Tamara now confesses she usually gets so angry that she destroys whatever her

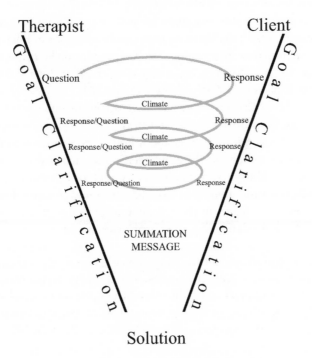

FIGURE 2. Therapist–client exchange during therapy.

husband brings home and throws it around the house. On occasion she has aimed at him and hit him. In answer to whether she thinks her temper affects the relationship, Tamara says that her husband's behavior exacerbates it but it has been a problem for her since she was a child.

This interaction illustrates how clients often begin to offer more information in the context of the emotional climate that can lead to a more clearly focused path to solution.

DUAL-TRACK THINKING

In an effort to understand and make the best use of clients' "unique way of cooperating," it is important for therapists to have a way of separating their own experience of clients' words and actions from the clients' description or display of them (Rober, 1999). This process requires awareness of our bodily reactions as well as our thoughts. (Andersen, 1995; Johnson, 1987). Such awareness of one's reactions in relation to clients has a cumulative effect. The more we practice it the better we get at it. Yvonne Dolan (1991) suggests that it means that "one is continuing to grow as a person and as a therapist" (p. 271).

One way to do this is to run two tracks in your mind simultaneously. One monitors the client and the other your own reactions. The client track picks up information about how to cooperate with the client (i.e., manner of speech, world view, beliefs, interactional style with you and others, and idiosyncratic manners of speech or metaphors). The personal track transmits our own thoughts, feelings, emotional reactions, hunches, and knowledge. In the case of a new client with whom one has yet to establish a relationship the client track might be:

> "This man is really scrutinizing the office and me. His facial expression is so tight. No smiles. He is really well groomed. He wears very expensive clothes. He offers just as little information as he can, and always with a sarcastic twist. Always using expressions like 'my staff,' 'my secretary,' 'my employees.' "

The personal track might simultaneously be noting:

> "His way of scrutinizing the office and me with that expression on his face make it seem like he's looking down his nose at everything. A little inappropriate on a Saturday morning to be dressed so formally. He wants me to know he's got an important position. This man makes me feel uncomfortable. I feel like he's testing me. I feel intimidated."

Reactions and judgments picked up on the personal track, regardless of how negative they may be, should not be suppressed. They are valuable because they warn us to be careful about our reactions. Without that warning we have much less of a chance to react sensitively to our clients. An inappropriate negative reaction can shame or alienate, and that is detrimental to the emotional climate. Thus, in the foregoing scenario, the therapist can respond to his reactions to the client by telling himself:

> "I'm the therapist and the client is probably intimidated. His demeanor and appearance may be his way of dealing with his anxi-

ety about coming. He may think I'll be critical of him because of his marital problems. He came because his wife asked him to for the sake of their relationship, so he's hurting. I must make him feel more comfortable."

The best way to maintain this distance from personal feelings toward clients is to call on the theoretical assumptions. For example, in this case *every client is unique* could help one to focus on the individuality of the client, and deliberately question him about his work and its importance. This is likely to reduce his anxiety and need to act in an overbearing manner. Similarly, *emotions are part of every problem and solution* could lead to the recognition that this client is uncomfortable in the situation and serves to distract from one's own emotions.

Another situation in which dual-track thinking is useful occurs when a client reveals that he or she has done something, or intends to do something, of which we really disapprove. In such a case, our personal track can prevent us from showing or expressing disapproval and can remind us that our job is to help people make good decisions for themselves. For example, the assumption *You can't change clients; they have to change themselves* guides us toward questions that help clients weigh the advantages and disadvantages of their own decisions.

It is just as important to use dual-track thinking to process our positive reactions and responses to clients as to use it to process our negative ones. Inappropriately positive responses can make a client feel patronized. If our personal track is registering that a compliment, or positive reframe, is far-fetched it is best not given.

Dual-track thinking also provides important information for composing the summation message. This is discussed in Chapter 6.

CASE EXAMPLE: LAURA

The following case example illustrates the various aspects of the therapist–client relationship that were discussed earlier, with a particular emphasis on how to stay with the client and be positive at the same time

Laura was a 45-year-old freelance graphic artist. At the time she came to see me she had been divorced for 10 years. She had two daughters, ages 18 and 22. The older one was out of the home. Laura had a live-in partner for the past 8 years, Sam. She began to present her problem as soon as she sat down, and before I had a chance to start socializing. Anxious clients sometimes do that and for the sake of the emotional climate it is best to cooperate. Missing information can always be filled in later.

LAURA: The problem as I see it . . . well, I recently read Bradshaw's *Healing the Shame That Binds You* [1988] and I really related to some of what he was saying. I feel I've come up against a new level of issues in my life, I guess, and that looked like a good explanation to me. There's a really scared little kid in me that's being challenged more than she is capable of dealing with . . . (*starts to cry*) I'm feeling really sad. [To convey understanding I said that she sounded frightened as well as scared. She nodded and continued.] I've been experiencing depression since last fall—not very long—not very deep—24 to 36 hours—that scares me. I've healed a lot in my life. I didn't expect this to happen—to feel so powerless. That's traumatic! I've even had some academically suicidal thoughts.

I felt somewhat overwhelmed by this dramatic presentation but had to interrupt to clarify the suicidal thoughts. I asked what "academically suicidal thoughts" meant and Laura explained that they were thoughts such as "I can understand why people want to kill themselves when they feel like this all the time." However, she said she actually couldn't do it because she believes in reincarnation.

Nevertheless, I did a suicide assessment during which Laura said, "I can't imagine taking a gun to my head, or taking pills or mutilating my body; I'd never do anything like that. I hate blood and gore and all that stuff. I'm just concerned whether I could get detached enough from my body to do something like that."

Once again, to be certain that I understood, I asked for clarification of "getting detached from her body." Laura did not seem to have a clear idea of what exactly she was afraid of. She did not recall ever having experienced anything that remotely felt like being dissociated or detached even when she meditates, which she does regularly. I moved on by reflecting that it must be scary not to feel in control and decided that there did not seem to be any risk of her hurting herself at this time.

Laura continued for a while to describe her feelings in a diffuse manner. Her speech was pressured and she seemed to be getting more upset. I thought it might be more helpful to her to help her clarify how she will know she is feeling better than to continue in this manner.

LAURA: I'll feel better when I have more enthusiasm for life . . . when I feel like some of it is fun rather than work. It feels so hard and stressful. [This answer was too vague for me once again.]

THERAPIST: What areas of life in particular?

LAURA: Mostly in relationship to socializing and work, not family relations or intimate relations.

THERAPIST: Socializing means friends? [I did not want to move on until I was perfectly clear about what Laura meant.]

LAURA: Yes. You see, I'll know I'm better when I can appreciate what is going right in my life—what's easy and fun—I get hung up on what is hard and what is not working.

THERAPIST: So what is usually easy and fun? [Notice the focus on the positive side of the statement.]

Laura listed her relationship with her partner and with her older daughter. She also said that she did not have material needs and that she had a budding graphic design business she enjoyed.

Hoping to continue in a more focused manner, I asked Laura a scaling question to help her evaluate the good in her life in relation to the bad, but she ignored me and went into a complaint about how the better she does professionally she more scared she gets.

Here is an example of the benefit of dual-track thinking. My personal track was registering that Laura wanted to complain more than work on solutions, so it was better not to ask more about positive exceptions. However, on the personal track I argued that her diffuse complaints were probably more harmful than helpful because they seemed to increase her anxiety. Therefore, I chose to ask a scaling question, hoping that its relative view might be helpful to Laura.

THERAPIST: So, overall, what percentage of daily living is comfortable as compared to stressful for you on a daily basis?

LAURA: It's 70% stressful. [Her way of cooperating was to be negative.]

THERAPIST: Daily?

LAURA: Yes.

THERAPIST: Around work and socializing . . . or just socializing? [I was checking out whether this was in agreement with what Laura had said earlier.]

LAURA: No . . . just about how to run my life—keeping the house clean, going shopping. [This was inconsistent with what she said before, but I decided to ignore that because it would only divert from focus.]

THERAPIST: So, what is different during the 30% of times when things aren't so stressful?

LAURA: (*ignoring the question*) I have a lot of options and I can't decide which are right for me or not!

My personal track registered that Laura wanted to be negative and that I better watch the emotional climate. I noted that *therapists cannot change clients; clients can only change themselves.* Therefore, I began to listen more carefully. Laura explained that when Bradshaw talks about fear of abandonment he relates it to inadequate bonding in early years that prevents the formation of proper limits in later life. She saw this as a reason for getting lost in making decisions about her many opportunities.

There are two reasons why some solution-focused therapists might choose not to follow Laura's train of thought at this point: (1) It is theoretically incongruent to explore this type of causality; and 2) if one chooses to respond to this type of causality to stay where the client is, it will take the client into past, negative territory. On the other hand, not cooperating with Laura could make her feel abandoned once again.

So I continued to listen to the complaints.

As I listened I became aware I was feeling uncomfortable. In checking that out with myself I noted that the session was coming to an end and all Laura had gotten out of it was the opportunity to complain. That might be useful, but she seemed to get more and more agitated as the session went on. I believed that it might be therapeutic if she left with a little more clarity about the direction of therapy. I was going to look to her for an answer to that, but first I had to make certain that I had understood her correctly

THERAPIST: Well, it sounds like there are many things on your mind that are making you feel very sad and confused. You've told me that you feel out of control at times and that you have fears about failing. You are very stressed, you have had academic suicidal thoughts, and there are questions about inadequate bonding and abandonment that may be an issue. That's a lot to deal with. I was just wondering, if I had a magic wand right now and could make anything happen overnight that you would want to have happen, what would things be like for you when you wake up to tomorrow morning? [There are many different ways to ask the miracle question. The objective is to get the client to imagine a solution.]

LAURA: I'd have a goal, a good picture of where my life is heading.

THERAPIST: What do you think that goal will be? [The future tense is deliberate. It suggests the therapist's attitude about the possibility of change.]

LAURA: A sense of comfort with myself. A clear picture of what I can and cannot do. I'd have a sense of integration that tells me who I am, and that I will stay that way. [Once again Laura changed the description of her goal, but this time I became aware that a theme had developed: a search for identity. I decided to ask for exceptions in that area, using her language.]

THERAPIST: Have there been times when you have felt that integration?

Laura gave examples of business achievements and childrearing. She was unable to describe what made her feel integrated in those situations. I wondered whether it may have something to do with meeting goals she had set for herself? Laura said yes, particularly with regard to her older daughter. She was launching her and developing a healthy adult relationship with her as planned. (I consider it appropriate to offer ideas to clients as we explore their solutions. Questions are not the only way to interact with clients. However, ideas are always presented tentatively, so clients can reject them without a sense of disagreement.)

No sooner did Laura begin to talk about her positive relationship with her older daughter than she shared her concerns that her younger daughter, who was about to leave home, might not fare as well.

LAURA: I feel pressure on myself that this is the test of all my parenting, so that gets kind of scary.

THERAPIST: Sounds like with her leaving you feel like you are about to get a report card!

Laura laughed and nodded. Laura said that she had always worried about this daughter because the daughter resembles her so much in every way. When Laura was her daughter's age she was "very messed up" but no one knew it. Laura's parents believed her to be doing well in college when she was actually into drugs and alcohol and had to have an abortion and was very depressed.

LAURA: I was hurting so badly during those years. What if my daughter is hurting like that and not able to communicate with me?

I felt like I was at a decision point again. Should I stay with Laura's concerns about her daughter or continue to help her clarify a focus for therapy? Because time for the interview was almost up, I opted to do both.

THERAPIST: So you achieved your goal with your older daughter, but you are now concerned whether you will succeed with the younger one. That's understandable because you think she resembles you so much. I can see where you would want a better connection with her than you had with your parents. But how else will my magic wand make a difference tomorrow morning?

LAURA: I'll welcome challenges. Perhaps I'd live in a different place, build a house. I'd like to think about that with enthusiasm instead of thinking it is too much work.

Laura went on to say that had been in therapy on and off for the past 12 years since she left her husband. Her decision to leave him came when she felt she had had enough of not being herself. At that point she began to grow and was relatively happy, with occasional peaks and valleys, unlike the extreme feelings she was having now.

THERAPIST: How did you manage to keep it from getting to that extreme stage then? [Always search for past resources.]

LAURA: I didn't expect as much of myself. . . . I was just starting out. I also had a lot of support. I went to groups, had more friends than I have now. I am also more isolated since I freelance than when I worked for someone else.

THERAPIST: How will you know you have achieved what you want now?

LAURA: When I'm more relaxed.

THERAPIST: How will you recognize that? What will you notice about yourself, and others notice about you when you are more relaxed?

LAURA: I'd feel more confident in my decisions—not stupid and irrational.

THERAPIST: Tell me about times in your life when you felt confident.

LAURA: When I made my decision to be with Sam.

THERAPIST: How did you make that decision?

LAURA: (*beginning to brighten noticeably and slowing down her speech*) I listened to myself about what I need physically and emotionally, my gut feelings.

THERAPIST: Are you usually right about your decisions?

LAURA: Yes, except in the last 5 months.

Laura then confessed feeling she made a mistake by pushing her younger daughter to start packing for college too soon. She had wanted to avoid stress in the last minute. When she kept nagging about it her daughter finally got angry and told her to stop making her so nervous about leaving. Subsequently, her daughter came down with mononucleosis, postponing her departure for another month.

LAURA: (*with tears in her eyes*) I should have known better.

Laura reverted to complaints, particularly about her business. I was concerned that my attempts to focus her might have been detrimental to the emotional climate. To remedy this I just sat back and listened empathically while Laura vented more about the depth of her depression.

LAURA: The feelings I have lately are "off the charts" for me, more like something I would associate with a big loss, like her father dying.

THERAPIST: Do you think your last child leaving home may represent a big loss? [The offer of an idea the client may not have or be aware of having is a perturbation.]

LAURA: Well, I didn't think so!

THERAPIST: It is the end of an era for you. You put so much effort into parenting. Do you think this may be playing a role in your feelings of depression?

LAURA: (*silently thinking for about a minute*) Yes, I do.

The decision I now had to make was whether or not to respond in the direction of the loss and grief. Laura's presentation had been so emotional all along that I though a cognitive perturbation might be more helpful for her. Therefore, I asked an advantage question that would offer her a both–and perspective.

THERAPIST: I just had another thought. . . . This may sound like a strange question, and I want to assure you that I understand how depressed you feel about all the things you have told me, and how much you are suffering, but I was wondering if you think there might be any advantage to . . . anything positive about the way you have been feeling instead of being enthusiastic, decisive and full of life?

LAURA: (*silent again for a long time; suddenly*) It's a form of protection, to keep me from having too much responsibility. (*Looks startled.*) I don't know where that came from?

THERAPIST: Why now?

LAURA: I don't know. Well, maybe . . . my thought is with the kids leaving I could leave.

THERAPIST: Leave? . . . Milwaukee? Sam? [I was surprised by this answer. I had to understand it before I moved on.]

LAURA: Both.

THERAPIST: Is that something you have been conflicted about?

Laura explained that she has never been on her own. She had gone from her parents' home to a dorm at college to marriage. After her divorce she had to care for her children.

LAURA: Part of me feels like I'll have no strings for the first time.

THERAPIST: That can feel scary as well as good!

Laura explained that she really didn't want to leave Sam but in order to feel that she is continuing to grow she will have to experience herself as more emotionally and financially independent of him. She seemed to believe that this was an either–or situation and I responded by exploring the both–and.

THERAPIST: Can you imagine feeling both more independent and still attached at the same time? Or does it have to be one way or the other?

Laura thought she didn't know because she tended to either overconform or rebel. She believed that she stores up resentment and when she gets really angry she explodes, even at work.

LAURA: I'm better than I used to be but I still need to learn more about how to be myself in a system—that's why I isolate myself.

I became aware that I felt frustrated because Laura moved into self-criticism again. *Solution-focused therapy goes slowly* popped into my mind and I made no further attempts at solution talk.

THERAPIST: Well, I can see there is a lot going on for you that you need to talk about. I didn't get a chance to tell you when we started, but I will be taking a short break to think about what we talked about and to tell you what I think, and maybe make a suggestion.

I was working alone without a team, so I left the therapy room and went to my office to think and formulate a summation message (see Chapter 7). This is the message I read to Laura after the break:

THERAPIST: What I heard you tell me today is that you have had a difficult life, one in which you did the right things expected of you all the time and tried to please, but gradually, over the past 10 years or so you have begun to find more of a balance between pleasing others and doing what is right for you. You also told me that you have overcome a lot of difficult situations in your life like drug and alcohol abuse, an unsuccessful marriage, raising children by yourself, and you have healed and grown a lot. You said you have come now to work on issues that you think are connected with excessive depression, particularly issues of abandonment. You also shared that your younger daughter, who you think is a lot like you, is preparing to leave home. Naturally you are concerned whether you have done a good job raising her or whether she is happy or unhappy as you were at this point. Her leaving puts you on the brink, for the first time in your life, of being able to say to yourself, "I can just please myself. I have no one to be responsible to or for." (*asking Laura to confirm that I had understood her*) Did I get that right? (*Laura nods.*) My response to what you told me is that it takes a lot of intelligence and strength to grow as much as you have. While you have reached a good point in life to be at, and you should give yourself credit for it, it is also a period of loss and uncertainty. It makes sense that you would feel sad because a phase of life is ending and excited, and scared, because a new one is beginning. It isn't at all unreasonable to feel emotionally out of control and immobilized at times like that. Especially for someone like you who has put a lot of effort into trying to understand herself and have a grip on life.

You know, dependence/independence isn't a matter of either–or. To be truly independent one knows when to ask for help and when to take care of oneself. You seem to know this already, because you understand the value of support and also reached out by coming here. (*Laura nods.*) Do you have any comments? (*Laura shakes her head no.*) Well, I'm wondering whether you want to come back again to talk to me?

LAURA: Oh, yes, definitely. You seem to understand.

THERAPIST: Then something you may want to think about for next time is, "When I am ready to move ahead with my life, how can I do that gradually without feeling I am abandoning anyone or that I am being abandoned? [Notice that I returned to her original theme of abandonment.]

LAURA: I like what you said about dependence and independence! I know I don't want to be alone, but how can I be in a relationship and be more myself?

When Laura came back to see me 10 days later she seemed like a different person. She was smiling and focused. She reported having had a challenging time since she saw me but that she felt in control.

LAURA: I stayed with myself and trusted that everything will be OK. My assignment zeroed in on what I had been thinking too, and your understanding it said to me it made sense to you, too . . . that we are on the same track. Then I realized that a big part of being afraid of being abandoned is staying with myself and not abandoning myself . . . not getting so emotional and staying with the situation . . . to stay calm within myself.

THERAPIST: How do you keep from abandoning yourself?

LAURA: Remind myself there is a "me." There is someone here inside of me to stay with. Some of the isolation I felt recently was that I wanted feedback so much from others I went too far toward them and couldn't hear myself. My past self has been functioning well overall for a long time.

Laura then shared that she was tired of taking care her of her daughter—she needed time away from her—and that she had been very upset at the thought that she might not leave home now as planned. However, since the last session she had realized that it is only a matter of a time, and that this short delay offers them a chance to separate well. She also reported having gotten a new design project that excited her.

At the end of the session Laura asked whether she needed to keep seeing me. I said she was the best judge of that. She made another appointment for a month later with the agreement that if she did not feel she needed it she would cancel. She did cancel it. I happened to run into Laura a couple of times since then and she reported that she continues to do well.

I chose to talk about Laura because she represents the type of person who is particularly challenging to solution-focused therapists. It is a struggle to decide how long to cooperate with the negativity and if and when to try to divert the client toward positives and the future. The answer is usually a mixture of both, depending on the client's responses. The important thing is to put more value on the evolving relationship and the emotional climate than on the use of technique. This is confirmed by a study of the relational process of SFT (Beyerbach et al., 1996), which found that therapists' attempts to control the conversation with clients to produce change (e.g., by a pattern of frequent questions and answers) results in a higher premature dropout rate for clients. The researchers suggest that just listening to clients at times without intervening can be beneficial in the long run.

In this case, the conversation during the session must certainly have conveyed an effort on my part to understand, but Laura's responses during the session suggested she may have wondered whether I did. Laura's comments after I read the message verified that she felt affirmed and had gotten a new perspective. I believe it is the summation message that provided the trust that solidified Laura's relationship with me.

In the next chapter I continue to talk about the choices therapists have to make in relation to clients, but more for the purpose of deciding what to respond to and what to ignore.

3

Understanding Clients

A common question asked by solution-focused therapists is how to determine what to respond to and what to ignore when talking with clients. It does take a lot of experience to notice that clients have their own ideas about what they want to talk about and that they do not always answer our questions. To ignore their needs can sometimes have worse consequences than to force the conversation toward positives and the future because of the effect this pressure can have on the emotional climate. Yet the whole point of SFT is to have clients develop a different way of perceiving their situation. This chapter addresses the dilemma and offers suggestions on how to deal with it.

HEARING VERSUS LISTENING

The decision about what to respond to and what to ignore concerns the distinction between "hearing" and "listening." What we hear is everything our clients tell us. What we listen for is determined by our theory and its assumptions and refers to being alert for appropriate questions and responses (Lipchik, 1988a; Lipchik & de Shazer, 1986). For example, we know that presession change can be important for solutions (Weiner-Davis, de Shazer, & Gingerich, 1987) so we listen for it. Because we assume *nothing is all negative* when a client describes a particularly hopeless situation, we listen for any small detail that can be highlighted as an exception or strength. We do not ignore anything we hear, but at the same time, we only respond to what is potentially useful for the client. "Hearing" serves as a backdrop to listening and is a more passive process. What we hear builds a general awareness of what clients want and how they cooperate. It registers what they mean, what they may be feeling, and what they are not saying. Sometimes we ask for clarification about what we hear because we get a clue that more clarity might facilitate a solution. This clarification may lead to a shift in direction, if the client agrees, and it then becomes the focus of our listening. As solutions become clear, listening to reinforce change may come to the forefront.

For example, if Zak's parents, referred by the guidance counselor of the local junior high school, come to consult me about Zak's uncontrolled aggression at school, I may also "hear" about his poor sleeping habits, his poor hygiene, and his bad relationship with his younger brother. I will ask the parents which problem they want to address first. If they decide to talk about Zak's relationship with his brother, that will be the focus of what I will be listening to. I cannot respond to everything the parents say because the conversation will be unfocused and the clients are likely to leave feeling more confused than when they came. Therefore, if, while listening, I hear the parents disagree about the cause for Zak's behavior toward his brother, I will ignore that at first, because *there is no true cause and effect in human behavior.* However, if I hear the disagreement as a distracting buzz to the conversation, I will begin to listen to it for signs of agreement between the parents that might be a step toward a solution. If, as I listen for agreement, I hear the disagreements between them go beyond Zak's problems, and parenting issues in general, I will ask the parents whether they want to talk about their general disagreements or Zak's relationship with his brother. If I do not make that clear I will not know what to respond to and what to ignore. This process of focusing the conversation was described earlier in a formulaic manner, but in actual practice it can be contextualized with understanding and empathy to establish a secure emotional climate.

MEANING

Hearing and listening are an integral part of language in the sense that they are a recursive process of coordination of linguistic interactions (Maturana, 1987, p. 211) with clients. We hear, and listen for the meaning our clients ascribe to what they tell us about their lives because it helps us understand their particular world view. While their meaning is subjective it is also "context dependent" (Anderson, 1997, p. 206). For example, the word "divorce" may have different meanings to a devout

Catholic and to an agnostic, to someone whose parents were divorced and to someone whose parents are happily married, to someone who has been through a previous divorce and to someone who has not. On one hand, our clients and we understand the definition of the word "divorce" in our society; on the other hand, we cannot assume to know the meaning the process of getting a divorce has for a particular client. It can mean failure, shame, sin, or relief.

For narrative therapists (Freedman & Combs, 1996; White, 1995; White & Epston, 1990), questions about meaning have the purpose of helping clients reflect on the stories about their lives and their relationships, and to consider and experience different ones that will be less problematic for them.

For the collaborative language systems therapist (Anderson, 1997; Hoffman, 1990, 1998), the entire therapy conversation is considered a way to generate new meanings that lead to "self-agency and problem dissolution" (Anderson, 1997, p. 109).

In SFT, inquiries about meaning provide our clients and us with more clarity about how the problem is perceived and how clients will know it is solved. For example, when a client who has a tempestuous relationship with her sister says she has come for help to "deal with the situation," it is necessary to ask what "dealing with the situation" means to her. It could mean that she wants to change something about herself or that she wants to change her sister. The difference can lead to different conversations about solution. Unless we are persistent about clarity we may end up having conversations about different topics.

Questions about meaning often lead to an answer that concerns emotions. If they do not, and it seems appropriate, they can be followed up with a question that elicits emotions. For example, if the foregoing client says she wants to change her sister so the sister does not talk in a demeaning way about her to their mother, this is an unrealistic goal because we cannot change someone else's behavior. However, asking how her sister's behavior affects her emotionally may prompt her to talk about feeling angry, rejected, or frightened, which can redefine the problem to one that has a more realistic solution because it requires her, not her sister, to do something different.

My description of how meaning should be used in SFT may sound purposeful, or strategic. Indeed, I intend to say that there is purpose and strategy to how we choose what to respond to and what to ignore (Quick, 1994). The decisions are based on our theory and information obtained from responses to questions determined by that theory. It is our intention that is of ultimate significance. The decisions we make in relationship to clients must be motivated by the genuine belief that *we cannot change clients; they can only change themselves,* and for the purpose of helping clients discover their own solutions.

Intentional inquiries about meaning just for the purpose of generating new meaning are not in keeping with solution-focused thinking even though they have the potential of generating information. Random questions about meaning can diffuse the solution-focused process rather than keeping it focused on solution.

PROBLEM TALK VERSUS SOLUTION TALK

One of the beliefs about SFT has been that "problem talk" should be ignored in favor of "solution talk." The terms "solution talk" and "problem talk" were coined at the Brief Family Therapy Center many years ago (de Shazer, 1994, p. 80) for clients' descriptions of the negative aspects (problem oriented) and positive aspects (exceptions, resources, recent changes) of their lives.

The effect of solution talk on clients has been documented by two research studies. Gingerich, de Shazer, and Weiner-Davis (1988) found that change occurs sooner, and therapy is shorter, when the therapist initiates solution talk as early as possible in the first session. Shields, Sprenkle, and Constantine (1991) found that treatment is more likely to be continued and be completed when solution talk is initiated early. This information is useful but must not be misinterpreted to mean that the therapist has to be directive at all times. The choices therapists make in relation to clients must be based on each individual situation, with the quality of the therapist–client relationship always the utmost consideration.

Clients, not therapists, determine whether they want to talk about solutions. Laura, whose case was described in Chapter 2, kept returning to problem talk whenever solution talk was raised, even after a few positive responses. Her reactions suggested that she needed to talk about her problem. However, as noted, the forays into future talk may have registered anyway and indirectly facilitated the solution Laura found for herself between sessions. We never know how what we say affects our clients, even when they do not respond, but it is safer to follow their lead than to push too hard in a direction they do not want to go.

Marilyn LaCourt, one of the original codevelopers of SFT, has developed the term "transition talk" for the phase during which the therapist communicates hope, assesses motivation, focuses on small changes, and identifies past successes. She believes that problem talk is not necessarily negative because it is an opportunity to communicate understanding and empathy, prioritize complaints, and clarify what the client wants (personal communication, 1999).

The danger of using descriptive terms such as "problem talk" and "solution talk" is that they are very concrete (either–or) and can lead us toward being too directive with our clients. Aside from the effect on the emotional climate, such labels can prevent us from both hearing and listening for other subtleties that could be valuable for solutions. Rather than thinking of "problem talk" and "solution talk" it is better to think of the conversations we have with clients as an interactional process ("languaging"). During this process, the problem and possibilities for solutions are gradually woven into a fabric that will represent the solution to the client in the end. It is the meaning people ascribe to a situation that defines it as a problem or a solution, not the words used to describe it. Feeling sad can be considered a problem if it is believed to be a disease, or a solution if it means that a person who has avoided grieving is finally accepting a loss.

Labeling any aspects of our conversations with clients has little value and can be distracting. If we are intent on hearing what clients are saying, regardless of whether their words are negative or positive, we will understand when to begin listening for an opportunity to help clients achieve another perspective. For example, a client may be describing a problem and may suddenly use the past tense: "I'm having such a hard time getting myself going in the morning because I sleep so badly, and I have such bad dreams. I take such a long time to get out of bed. I used to fall back asleep several times, but I still don't get up as quickly as I should." Notice the client said "used to" fall back asleep. This may be a positive seed that should be cultivated. First, the therapist can try to communicate understanding for how badly the client feels about the situation and then he or she may ask, "Did I hear you say there is a change in your waking pattern in the morning lately?" If the client says yes, it may offer an opportunity to discuss what that change may mean, how it happened, whether the client wants it to continue to happen or make it happen more often or differently. This gradual elaboration on a word in the past tense cushioned in an emotional climate of acceptance and understanding has the potential of helping the client think, act, and feel differently about his or her situation than he or she did before that conversation.

The artful task of the therapist is to tailor the therapeutic process to individual clients. This task calls for intuition and judgment that is honed by experience. The bottom line is that we tailor the therapeutic process based on how well we hear and understand our clients' particular way of experiencing their world.

CONTENT VERSUS PROCESS

The family therapist talks with the family about the content
of the problem but thinks about the process of discussion
by which they try to solve it.
—NICHOLS AND SCHWARTZ (1995, p. 487)

Content is what clients tell us about their situations; process is how clients act in relation to what they say. Clients are not usually aware of their process. An extreme example might be a family that talks about serious, life-threatening problems in a lighthearted, teasing manner, with lots of laughter.

Attending to process has fallen out of favor since therapists have turned from systems thinking, which focused on behavior, to language, which focuses on cognition. Interrupting patterns of behavior has been replaced by creating new meaning. Instead of asking, "What does Mother do when Father yells at Johnny for spilling the milk?", we are now inclined to ask what Dad's yelling about spilled milk means in terms of Mom and Dad's relationship, and their relationship with Johnny.

However, if we think of language as an action, and therapy as having the goal of changing action (behavior, cognition, and emotions), then process is still relevant. The only difference is that we are no longer just interested in observable behaviors but also in the emotional aspects of the process.

The goal of SFT is to use language with clients in a way that affects content and process, much like strategic therapists do. However, this can rarely be accomplished by techniques alone. To achieve this goal requires therapists' being attuned to how clients cooperate both in terms of what they say and how they act.

I would like to clarify that when I talk about process I am referring to how clients act toward each other, as well as to how therapists interact with clients. Our process with clients is a conversation in which they tell us and show us how they are stuck, and we talk with them about their past, present, and future ideas and experiences about being un-stuck. However, that conversation has to be conducted in a manner that fits the clients' world view and interactional style, such as being detail oriented, controlling, artistic, competitive, or conforming. That type of conversation creates a new process that is more likely to lead to a solution.

The urgency to divert clients' conversations toward behavioral descriptions can result in impasse. Our clients' process involves emotions as well as behaviors even though they may not be as easy to observe. The cold, detached behavior of a husband does not mean he is not hurting as much as his hysterical, clinging wife and that that pain does not affect his process as much as hers. Therefore, I am suggesting that therapists deliberately touch on feelings with all clients because the feelings are inseparable from behavior and cognition. There is some evidence, in fact, that emotions are an overriding force in behavior (LeDoux, 1996; Panksepp, 1998). We need little scientific proof that they are central to couple and family relationships.

Mary, an attractive 35-year-old woman, came to therapy to figure out what is wrong with her because she could not sustain relationships with men. She reported that she went to singles dances hoping to meet men, and they always lost interest in her after the first dance. Occasionally a man would ask her out on a date, but he would never call back for a second invitation. She did not understand this because she felt she was not unattractive or dumb, she had a good job, and she tried to be pleasant.

Mary could not come up with any exceptions to her complaints. A miracle would mean that someone would find her interesting enough to want to spend lots of time with her and eventually marry her. No one ever wanted to spend more time with her after a date or two. She had no idea what she would have to do differently to get a man to call her again. Mary had no idea about her process. Asking her about what these rejections meant to her would likely draw her further into berating herself. It is self-evident that Mary thought her problem was that she was deficient in some manner.

Circular questions (Selvini Palazzoli, Cecchin, Prata, & Boscolo, 1978) had a good chance of shedding some light on Mary's process so she could consider some different options. For example: "What do you think men would say about how you react when they flirt with you?"; "How do you want men to perceive you?"; "How would you feel if they perceived you that way?"; "How do you think that would make a difference?"; "What do you think you have to do to make men think you are interested in them?"; "What do you notice about women who seem to hold men's interest?"

The solution-focused techniques did not fit Mary because they lacked a context in which she could consider them. Mary was only able to perceive her situation in her own way and that is why she was stuck. Her view did not consider the perspective of the men she wanted to attract. In that context she might be able to find a solution. The circular questions were an attempt to offer her that. There are clients who have a difficult time seeing things from any other perspective than their own. Presuming that Mary was not one of them, expanding her view to include process would offer her the opportunity to consider whether she has the ability, or the desire, to experiment with some changed behaviors toward men. If feelings do not come up naturally as part of such a conversation the therapist should ask about them. This will provide a much richer source of information to draw on for a solution. This therapeutic process will not, however, prolong therapy unnecessarily because it addresses emotions. Indeed, it may shorten therapy because of that.

The following case illustrates the process of making choices based on the various concepts described in this chapter.

CASE EXAMPLE: MARIE

Marie was a 26-year-old African American female, divorced, with two children, a 4-year-old girl and a 2-year-old boy. She was interviewed by a young man who recently entered a training program for SFT and was still struggling with what to respond to and what to ignore. The supervisor-in-training stressed trying to avoid problem talk and to get into solution talk as quickly as possible.[1]

THERAPIST: (*after some socializing and joining*) How are you hoping that we can help you?

MARIE: Oh, well . . . hmm . . . sometimes . . . they say it kind of helps mentally if you can talk to people and then sometimes you can't . . . and in my case, you know, <u>I keep everything bottled up inside, where it, you know, causes pain to me, nobody else but just pain to</u>

---

[1]Underlined portions of the dialogue indicate content that should be heard or listened to.

me, and they felt I should talk to someone. (*Starts right in to talk about her problem and the pain it causes her.*)

THERAPIST: Who's "they"? (*Ignores what he hears and asks about the referral source.*)

MARIE: The hospital. The doctor that I went to see.

THERAPIST: Is that a psychiatrist?

MARIE: No, it was a referral that they had to fill out and they suggested that I come here and talk out my problems.

THERAPIST: Um, I see. And did you agree with their suggestion? [Responded to what he heard by asking the client whether she agreed. This is a helpful way to getting an idea about her level of motivation.]

MARIE: Well, I thought about it and I said . . . OK!

(*The therapist and Marie both laugh.*)

THERAPIST: All right! And what are you hoping to see changed by coming here? [Moved right into solution talk to focus on a goal.]

MARIE: Well, I can't say right now. I don't know really. Just that I have things that've been bothering me and <u>I'm trying my best to really, like cope with it, but it just seems like there isn't any answer for me, no matter what I try to do. Nothing works if I try to make my life a little better than what it is, and that's my right, so I really don't know.</u>

THERAPIST: Is there one big thing that's bothering you or just a lot of little stuff?

Marie had hinted at unsuccessful attempts to improve her life. The therapist tried to focus her by asking her to categorize the problem as little or big rather than by asking for more clarification. To establish a good emotional climate and clarity it is best to use the client's own words in framing a question, particularly at the beginning of therapy. For example: "What is there no answer to in your life?" or "What are you trying to do that isn't working?"

MARIE: Well, mostly big, mostly little things. . . . I don't know, I just really don't know to exactly explain it.

THERAPIST: How have you been coping so far? [The therapist and the client were not on the same track. He attempted to look for exceptions about how she copes when she had not even begun to articulate her problem.]

MARIE: Well, most of the time instead of really getting out, I don't get out. I stay cooped up and most of the time I am just really by myself, and to be honest, just don't feel like being around anybody.

THERAPIST: Hmm. So what you have been doing to cope so far is to do what?

MARIE: Well I like to sit down and write or read a book or some of those things and then, it only passes the time sometimes, and that's about it. Most of the time I just don't know the answers.

THERAPIST: What do you think that the doctor was thinking that you should come for? [Attempted to get referral source's reason for sending client rather than continuing to understand her needs.]

MARIE: <u>He didn't want to talk to me.</u>

THERAPIST: Oh, yeah!

MARIE: Um. . . . It's puzzling because I said, now why would he suggest that I come to, like a therapy session. Wait a minute, <u>am I crazy or what?</u> Then he said no, no, it's just that sometimes it can help. Like I thought <u>maybe I was getting ready to go into one of them rages you know, or something like that,</u> but then it would be best because, you know, <u>I've been having like pains, like if I'm upset a lot then the whole entire body hurts, or I'll get them tension headaches</u> sometimes, like someone pounded you on your head and then at night when I go to bed, I don't go to bed till about 4:00 or 5:00 in the morning, then I'm up again.

THERAPIST: What time do you get up?

Marie told the therapist she was afraid she might have a deep-seated problem because of the doctor's attitude and her physical symptoms. Instead, the therapist asked about what time she got up. His choice could reinforce Marie's idea that there was something really wrong with her because this expert was not understanding her. Moreover, because Marie said the physician who referred her "didn't want to talk to her," the therapist should make a special effort to be different, that is, to connect with her and to be direct.

MARIE: I mean I really don't get that much rest. <u>I figure it must be something that is really bothering me that I just don't want to know, but then again, you know, it's like you really want to know.</u>

THERAPIST: Well, what has to happen in your mind for you to finish your session or your sessions here and to say to yourself, boy, that helped! What will have to happen at home with you? [Attempted to define a goal. The phrasing of the second question, "what will have to happen at home" limits Marie's possibilities for answers. The problem has not been defined enough yet to warrant the focus on the home.]

MARIE: Well, that's another tough one. I really don't know. (1) Like I said, it's some things that have been happening that, you know, shouldn't be happening and then there's people that, should be, or shouldn't be in my life, but then they keep constantly coming back in and out . . . (2) and then there's my mother. It's just very difficult, (3)you want to just get away with your kids and not let nobody know where you are. But then when you get a chance to do that(4)somebody is thinking you are different or weird just because you don't drink or do some of the things they do.

THERAPIST: Um, well, let me ask you another question. If you went to sleep tonight, sounds like you don't do that very much, but if you went to sleep tonight and you work up tomorrow morning and the problems were gone, they were solved, what will be different?

Notice that the client's previous answer contained four points: (1) Some people are coming in and out of her life who should not be; (2) her mother is a problem; (3) she wants to get away with her kids; (4) people see her as being "weird" if she doesn't behave like they do. This requires a response that tells the client she has been heard and that the therapist feels for her in her confusion and distress. For example: "You seem to be bothered by a lot of things. I'd like to hear more about them. Which one do you think you want to start with?" "It sounds like you people are critical of you when you make choices for yourself."

The therapist's choice to ask a miracle question may be his attempt to get an idea of what Marie wants. The miracle question can be a way to help clients clarify what they want.

MARIE: Well, mainly I would likely try to, you know, to better myself as a mother.

THERAPIST: OK.

MARIE: (continues) . . . and when you're used to being independent and you have to depend on somebody else, that can hurt.

THERAPIST: Are you used to being independent or dependent? [This would be a good place to ask the client about the meaning of those terms.]

MARIE: Well, sometimes one . . . sometimes another.

THERAPIST: If a miracle happened tonight and you woke up tomorrow and your problems were gone, which one would you be?

MARIE: Well, like I said that's confusing. I've sat down several times and debated whether if this was to change or that . . .

THERAPIST: If what was to change? [This is a good example of the therapist responding to what he heard and testing whether it is something to listen for more closely.]

MARIE: OK. I don't communicate with anybody, and I feel that if I could just get away from the surroundings that I'm in now, you know, I might do better, than again I can't really say whether I would, but I would feel more at ease . . . wouldn't have to be under so much stress.

THERAPIST: Ah, tell me, if that miracle were to happen, do you think you'd be alone less, you'd be around people a little more, communicate a little more?

Marie finally provided a clearer description of her problem. It might have been more effective at this point to ask the miracle question in a more open-ended manner: "If that miracle were to happen what will be different?")

MARIE: Um. . . . I don't know . . . I just can't, well, I never could, be around people that, you know, always want you to be the way they want you to be. . . . I figure, I can only be me and you can only be you, so if you can't accept that then that's fine.

The supervisor called in to remind the therapist to ask about the physical problems for which the client was referred.

THERAPIST: Well, seems these days you've been having these headaches and pains and people are coming in and out of your life. What about the times that you don't have headaches and that you feel OK about yourself? What's going on then? [Did not respond to what he heard and continued solution talk. Looking for an exception about one of multiple complaints that has not been selected by the client is usually not productive.]

MARIE: Well, not too much of anything. I mean, I'm almost in a trance. You don't want to say anything and it's like you really don't know what to say to anyone. <u>Now, it's not that I'm not getting along with my children, I get along fine with them.</u>

THERAPIST: You do? Great! I know a lot of mothers who say they are constantly having problems with their little kids. [Reinforced a strength, which is a good supportive response in any situation.]

MARIE: It's not the children, '<u>cause you know, I say that if I had to have children I would rather wait until after I finish high school to do the things that I want to do</u> and so it happened. . . .

THERAPIST: What happened? [Good clarification]

MARIE: I mean, I got pregnant and you know, here comes one kid after the other.

THERAPIST: [Ignored another negative direction and tried to stay with strengths.] So you're managing them OK these days, then?

MARIE: Yeah.

THERAPIST: How do you manage to keep that part of your life going so smoothly?

For the next few minutes Marie described all her efforts to be a good mother and to raise her children to be strong and intelligent. Then she became clearer about her problem.

MARIE: Yeah, <u>the problem is mostly my family. I'm not sure who . . . my mother, my brothers, my friends, my husband, my ex boy friend. He seems to appear out of nowhere, that's really upsetting me. I am trying to figure out where, where did you come from, what do you want? And my husband, he's not giving me much credit for being me, and I don't like those guys that really think that a female is really stupid,</u> 'cause the guy that I was going with before, the ex one I was talking about, I went with him for 10 years and it was like, all of a sudden, when I got married, to the children's father, it's like I was being threatened not to get married, and I said well, after all these years you didn't decide to marry me, so why you want to come in my life now?

THERAPIST: So you've got a boyfriend now who's coming in and out and that's kind of confusing?

MARIE: Yeah, that's confusing, and Eddie, my husband, from what I know, he might be going through something. He's been through a prior marriage and it's like this is my first time ever married so why give me a hard time because the first one didn't do whatever you expected her to do, so don't push it off on me.

The therapist and Marie were now on the same track. Positive reinforcement about the client's relationship with her children and some sense that she was being understood might have helped Marie feel safer to be more open or less anxious so she was thinking more clearly. Marie went on to say she had no hope for reconciliation. However, she did not believe in divorce for religious reasons. These men were the only two she had ever had in her life, but she felt each one of them was trying to hold her back from doing what she really wanted to do. She wanted to go back to school and "take up a good trade so that I might be able to help my children in the long run." When she discussed these dreams with her mother, her mother discouraged her and told her to wait. She had gotten information about how to get more education anyway, but no one wanted to help her with child care, and her husband told her a good mother stays home with her kids. For the time being Marie was educating herself by going to the library and checking our books.

THERAPIST: You're really motivated.

MARIE: But it's just like I said. You do all these things, but you know there must be something that's really, really bothering you. Why these people come around me, telling me maybe if you would lose just a little bit more weight you'd be all right. I'm like, ha, ha, why don't you lose some! And then, if you get smart with them, they tell you . . . you think you're so this . . . or so that. It's just too much, too much!

THERAPIST: So what are you doing to let that go in one ear and out the other?

The therapist and Marie were well connected during this part of the interview. The therapist presupposed strengths here in order to reinforce them.

Marie said she tried to block it out, but at night it bothered her more and she ended up getting only 1 hour of sleep. The therapist wondered whether getting more sleep would reduce the stress of the other problems.

MARIE: Well, I wish it were that way, but <u>then it would probably be something else</u>, you know.

THERAPIST: What do you mean? [Good example of the therapist hearing the client and attempting to understand]

MARIE: Like, <u>I'm living in my mother's house, and it's like everything I do I have to check with her</u>. And it's like you don't do this, you don't do that without her permission, and I would feel much better if I got out on my own.

THERAPIST: What would it take for you to do that?

Marie explained that she did not have enough money for a security deposit and she did not want to ask anyone for help. Her only income was her welfare check because her husband was not paying regular child support.

At this point it would have been useful to make an empathic statement and perhaps normalize Marie's physical and emotional stress. Instead, the therapist was thinking, *a small change can lead to bigger changes*, and tried to build on Marie's positive statements.

THERAPIST: Well, you know, it sounds to me like you've got some really good plans for what you want to do with your life, getting an education, meanwhile educating yourself, working with your children. What I'm wondering is, those are really big things and what's going to be the first small step that you'll need to take toward getting those bigger things?

MARIE: Well, <u>I should probably sit down and make me an outline, and say to myself, well, I guess I would have to interview babysitters you know</u>. I don't want nobody that's gonna be all rough and mean and do anything to my children. So when I get to that step, then I guess I will go to the next one. . . .

THERAPIST: What will be the next small step? [It would have been helpful here to elaborate more on the babysitting until it appeared possible for the client.]

MARIE: Well, the next one would be to <u>go to school, enroll myself and probably take some tests</u>.

Marie described how anxiety provoking that would be for her because she would worry whether she had passed and whether there would
be more tests to take, and how she would arrange a schedule for the children to be taken care of.

THERAPIST: Well, let's say in this next week, what's going to be just a
small sign to you that you are starting, at least to head in the direction of doing some things that you want to do?

Marie said that the first thing she would need would be to be alone
for a little while but that this is impossible because no one will watch the
children. She related that she got her driver's license last year and now
her brother sometimes let her take the car and take the kids for a ride
when he noticed her looking down. The therapist congratulated Marie
on her effort and success at driving and asked what else she had on her
list to be achieved.

MARIE: I put many things on the list but you see, I don't really go out as
far as doing anything because there is always someone, you know,
knocking you down. One thing that I learned that sometimes you
might have to just scoot away from it all and then another thing is
I'm scared if I moved away from my mother's house that my husband would really, really just flip out. That is the reason that I come
here tonight is partly because living in your mom's house and all of
that, that's the house I grew up in, I can't be me. It's just that
through the prior experiences that I had, I can't take another let-
down. I figure like this, I have something to do that's personal and I
don't want to say exactly what, but, it really makes me sick that if I
ever wanted to go out and date, which I doubt seriously, I couldn't
really do it because there is so many people thinking how I'm supposed to be and telling me in not a nice way.

THERAPIST: You haven't met a guy who has your kind of ideals. [Heard
the client and attempted to reflect some understanding.]

MARIE: That's right. So it's like the same old, you know, ritual and all of
this crap about you have to, just because your married, you have to
do this because you're my wife. At the time that I was with him it
was like it was always me, never him.

THERAPIST: Well, let me ask you one more question before I take time to
meet with the team. In this week to come, if you will take just a
small step in the direction you want, what would it be?

MARIE: Well, the next step is bowling.

THERAPIST: Bowling?

MARIE: I like to bowl. So I would probably go out and practice some bowling. [Seemed to have an understanding about how a small change could make a difference.]

THERAPIST: So if you were to go out bowling one time in the next week, that would be a sign that you are going in the right direction?

MARIE: Yeah, or getting out. I'm getting out.

The therapist excused himself and went to meet with the team that consisted of two other students and the supervisor. The supervisor had asked the students to list all the compliments they had for Marie and to think about a homework assignment.

This is the message the therapist read to Marie after the break:

THERAPIST: Well, we are truly impressed with the goals that you have set for yourself. You are obviously very willing to work to achieve your goals and you have a clear outline how to get there and what it takes to achieve what you want. I'm also struck with your good relationship with your kids. You just have a lot of patience and a lot of love for them. It shows real clearly. I was also struck with what drive you have inside yourself to better yourself. Going to the library and studying. And getting your license! I mean, you set that as a goal and you had a lot of drive to achieve that. It's just amazing considering all the difficulties and uncertainties in your life right now that you are able to do so much actually, and on 1 hour of sleep.

MARIE: Well, I don't know what it is!

THERAPIST: (continues) While you may not appreciate it, we are convinced that you're on the right track to achieving what you want to do. So, I want to leave you with a homework assignment.

MARIE: OK!

THERAPIST: What we'd like you to do in the week to come is to notice and keep a record of all the things that you will do that continue to move you in the direction you want to go.

MARIE: OK, no problem.

It is certainly easy to review a transcript or videotape and describe what one would have done differently in a situation. The transcript filters out a lot of nonverbal communication that can affect the process.

Marie was a difficult client to interview even for an experienced therapist because of her fragmented way of presenting her case. However, she is representative of clients who are confused and confuse us, or express themselves in ways that are difficult to understand. Notice how the exclusive focus on content seemed to confuse the conversation even more. If the therapist and supervisor would have considered the process they would not have been drawn into it and joined all the other people in Marie's life who did not understand her. In cases such as this, the best thing to do is to put "being solution focused" on the back burner and just to listen carefully to understand the client better.

This case illustrates that techniques do not have the power to work on their own. They must be used in the context of an understanding of what to respond to and what to ignore. It may seem unfair to have used the work of a student and a supervisor-in-training as an illustration, but the emphasis on technique versus hearing and listening is not uncommon and perpetuates a way of doing SFT that is not good therapy.

Marie did not return for further sessions. This is not surprising because she did not find the answer for which she was looking. Marie had probably come primarily for confirmation that she was not crazy. An added bonus would have been to find an understanding person to talk to. That she was on track about expecting change to happen slowly was evident from her statement that she wanted to begin with a chance to go bowling. The message at the end reflected positives while neglecting Marie's problems and concerns. To convey understanding it is always best to reflect both the positives and negatives. Too positive a message can be interpreted as lack of understanding or as patronizing.

The next chapter continues to elaborate on the role of emotions in the solution-focused therapeutic process.

4

Emotions in
Solution-Focused Therapy

I remember my first clinical supervisor, many years ago, repeating over and over again, "Stay with the feelings." Later, when I took training in family therapy, another supervisor kept saying, "Stay away from the feelings." Today, I tell trainees, "Don't ignore the feelings."

The emphasis or lack of emphasis on emotion in psychotherapy depends on theoretical orientation. My first supervisor was trying to get me to make clients more aware of their repressed feelings so they would develop insight. My family therapy supervisor was directing me to notice interactional patterns for the purpose of interrupting them. Today, I tell trainees not to ignore the feelings because they are important resources for solutions, just as thoughts and behaviors are.

There is no consensus about the definition of feelings, affect, and emotion, only a general understanding that "affect" refers to a reflexive reaction, controlled by the autonomous nervous system, whereas feelings are the awareness of what one is sensing. Awareness is obviously a cognitive function, and juxtaposing it with feelings calls to mind past academic disputes about whether emotions can occur prior to, and independently of, cognitive processes or whether all emotional responses are preceded by some basic cognitive process (Ekman, 1992; Lazarus, 1982; Mandler, 1984; Zajonc, 1984). Recent findings in neuroscience (Damasio, 1994, 1999; LeDoux, 1996) obtained with imaging technology that allows observation of brain functions has put this argument to rest, at least for the time being. These neuroscientific studies have provided evidence that cognition and emotion are separate but interacting brain functions mediated by separate but interacting brain systems (LeDoux, 1996, p. 69). Consequently, if emotions are "a biological dynamic" that determines actions (Maturana & Varela, 1987, p. 247) they can be understood to involve affect, feelings, cognition, and behavior.

This information allows for the speculation that an emotional response to a surprise party, if it could be examined in slow motion, could affect us like this: You enter a room and are startled by the shouts of the people there. They notice your body posture change, your face flush, and its expression change before you even become aware of it. (Think of how often people seem frozen for a moment or two when startled or surprised.) It becomes a feeling when you become aware that you are having a sensation. What the sensation means and how you are going to react to it is emotion. Emotion depends on many variables unique to genetic and social development and the context of the particular situation. You coordinate emotional experience linguistically by asking yourself, "What happened?"; "What does what just happened mean?"; "Does it mean the same thing to the people in this room?"; "What is the right response?" In other words, reasoning and the "emotioning" all take place together and they are language. You might feel genuinely happy about being surprised or annoyed because you do not like being caught off guard. If your emotional response is genuine pleasure you will express that more or less effusively depending on your unique affective style. If you are annoyed you will try to hide it by acting as if you were pleased because it is socially frowned upon to show disapproval when people have gone to great lengths to please you. However, your affect may give you away with subtle nonverbal cues, particularly to people who know you well.

Emotions occur in a social context. They are essential to our physical and mental health. Past research with young monkeys and infants has demonstrated that physical and emotional development is stinted in the absence of normal nurturing, such as being held (Harlow & Harlow, 1962; Spitz, 1951).

The developers of systemic therapy, the Mental Research Institute's brief therapy model and SFT were not oblivious to these facts. They, like other family therapists, understood that an emotional connection, or joining, is important for establishing the initial connection with clients when they begin therapy (Cade & O'Hanlon, 1993; Haley, 1976; Minuchin, 1974; Walter & Peller, 1992). Emotions were just not considered necessary for practice. In fact, they were considered a hindrance because the emphasis was on behavioral patterns that had the advantage of "simplicity, concreteness, and minimalization of presuppositons and inference" (Fisch et al., 1982, p. 11) and could be easily observed and tracked. Behavioral patterns were interrupted with cognitive "news of difference" (Bateson, 1979) geared to offer clients a different way to think about their problem, such as positive reframes of their negative problem descriptions or paradoxical interventions. At one point in history, SFT included clients' feeling states and physiological reactions, among other client descriptions considered important for designing interventions (de Shazer, 1985), but under the influence of linguistic philosophy on SFT emotions, behavior and cognition were melded into "language" and not discussed further in terms of practice. Though this is theoretically sound, it is too vague for good practice. The rest of this chapter explains my thoughts about this, particularly in relation to emotions.

EMOTIONS VERSUS BEHAVIOR

Solution-focused therapists have traditionally guided clients toward behavioral descriptions of their goals so they can track progress better, even though most clients describe their complaints in terms of feelings. The therapist's response does not have to be in either a behavioral direction or an emotional one. We can cooperate with clients and use their feeling words in conversation without sacrificing the benefit of more concrete signs of progress (Turnell & Lipchik, 1999).

Ramona came to therapy complaining, "I feel so down that I can't move." Traditionally, a solution-focused therapist would ask, "What are you doing, or not doing, that tells you you are feeling that way?" Ramona might answer, "I'm not going to work or I'm not getting dressed. " Here Ramona's feelings are used as stepping-stones to thinking about doing, not as a locus of attention themselves.

I find it more useful to allow clients to state their complaints in words about their feelings as much as possible. These feelings are accepted with empathic reflections such as the following: "That can be very discouraging!" or "What a terrible way to feel!" The client's feelings are explored further with questions such as the following, "What other feelings are you having as a result of this?" or "What does it mean to you that you are feeling so down?", to give the client the opportunity to clarify his or her complaint. This may open up new directions for solutions. For example, if Ramona ends up clarifying that her problem is that it frightens her to feel so low, her clarification offers the opportunity for asking, "What has been most helpful for you in the past to deal with fear?" Answers to this question are likely to be couched in behavioral terms ("I called friends," or "I turned on the TV") without the therapist's help. Another option is to continue by asking, "What is it you are afraid of?" If the answer is, "I'm incompetent, immature, mentally ill, or just like my mother," it can be followed by "What will convince you that your fears are not justified?" This question also has a good chance of producing behavioral answer and, if not, the therapist can always ask for small signs of behavioral change at the end of the session.

Consider what would happen if Ramona were asked a scaling question about her fear (Kowalski & Kral, 1989). After coming up with a number on a scale from 1 to 10 signifying how scared she is about the way she feels, Ramona's indication about how she will know she is just a little bit less scared will almost certainly be in behavioral terms (e.g., "I will bite my nails less," or "I'll brush my hair."

The point is that it may be in the clients' best interest to talk with them in their language, even if that is emotion, rather than risk that they do not feel understood.

USING EMOTIONS TO FACILITATE SOLUTIONS

Solution-focused therapists are accustomed to thinking about what to ask clients but not to thinking about what clients are feeling, or what they themselves are thinking and feeling in relation to clients. Expanding awareness to include these aspects can facilitate the development of solutions for clients.

Sometimes clients come in so emotionally overwrought that they cannot describe what they are feeling. We may need to help them clarify before they can establish goals and find solutions. A word of caution, however. It is important to go slowly and be sensitive to clients' verbal and nonverbal responses during this process. Clients' inability to know what they feel may have served a positive function for a long time, a way of protecting themselves from feelings they cannot bear. A sudden lifting of the veil can be more disturbing than helpful.

CASE EXAMPLE: BETTY

Betty was a client who was very upset but had to be helped to clarify her feelings. She was a 42-year-old, single woman self-referred because of episodic, uncontrollable crying spells. These spells had gradually increased over the past 4 months. Betty could not connect them with anything specific that was going on at work or in her private life. Betty had never been married, lived alone with two cats, and was not involved in a relationship with a man at the time. She had several close girlfriends with whom she socialized.

Betty had been working in the accounting department of a chain of fast-food restaurants for the past 5½ years and had been promoted three times since she started. Six months earlier she had been moved into a middle-management position, which required her to supervise and train staff. Betty was pleased with the new position and wanted to get control over her emotions so she could continue moving up the corporate ladder.

Betty did not wait for me to socialize or ask any questions. She blurted out her symptoms the moment she sat down and kept analyzing what might be causing them. I listened and made empathic reflections for a long time. Then I asked a miracle question as a way to help Betty think about what she wanted from therapy, but she did not respond. She continued to question her symptoms given that she liked the new challenges at work and did not feel overworked. I noticed myself thinking (dual-track thinking) that the session was too negative for too long and the client was going to leave feeling worse if I did not intervene, so I asked her how she would know the problem was solved. "I think there is no answer . . . maybe I have to quit . . . or learn not to take things to heart." I wondered what she meant by "taking things to heart" and she described her feelings of rejection when staff she trained left for higher-paying jobs outside her company.

THERAPIST: Oh, that must be hard.

BETTY: Yeah, it means I have to train more people and start all over again

THERAPIST: So things are in a constant flux for you?

BETTY: Yes, but I can also understand their leaving.

Betty shared her employment history. She had been working since age 16, starting with part-time jobs in high school. She had always gotten excellent evaluations and wanted to have control over her emotions so that she could continue her good record.

THERAPIST: Well, has there ever been a time before when you felt out of control emotionally?

BETTY: Partly, which I think is normal.

THERAPIST: Yes.

BETTY: I lost both my parents a long time ago, my father in an automobile accident and my mother to cancer, so at holidays, like Christmas . . . I'm not married and don't have any children . . . it's hard.

THERAPIST: Of course, that is certainly a reason to be sad.

BETTY: I feel the same way . . . but these episodes now have been going on for a few months, past Christmas.

THERAPIST: Well, does anything at work make you feel sad, or feel like a loss?

BETTY: Do you mean whether I feel that I'm going to lose my job?

THERAPIST: No, you said that you sometimes feel very sad at Christmas because you lost your parents. Is there anything going on a work that gives you a sense of loss. Perhaps losing people you have trained?

BETTY: (*surprised*) Very insightful. That very well could be!

THERAPIST: But what do you think?

BETTY: I don't know! (*Starts to cry.*) I don't know anything! All I know is that everything seems too much right now.

THERAPIST: That must be hard for someone as efficient and conscientious as you are.

BETTY: It's awful. I just want it to stop. I mentioned to my girlfriend that maybe I should quit, and she said maybe I have a problem with change. But, I think I'm actually looking for change, not trying to avoid it.

THERAPIST: Change of job?

BETTY: Yes, because I can't go on like this. This is all I think about.

THERAPIST: And when you are thinking about it, what are your thoughts about?

Betty described office politics that upset her at work. She expressed disappointment in her supervisor, a man to whom she has reported for 3 years. Two years ago she had complained about him because his lax work habits had begun to reflect badly on her work. Betty noticed that he was more conscientious after that, but about 6 months ago, he seemed to slack off again. With increased responsibilities in her new position, her supervisor's lack of support added a great deal of unnecessary stress, particularly around complaints from staff whom she supervised.

BETTY: Now I'm in a higher position and I sometimes mention something to him . . . and he does listen to me when I say something . . . then when I point something out to him that should be attended to for the sake of the whole department his favorite comment is, "Well, I have to find an appropriate time to bring that up." Well, I don't think you can wait for an appropriate time to address problems with an employee. What if he doesn't find an appropriate time for weeks or months. That's what usually happens. You take care of it right away! (*Her face is getting flushed and her voice sounds very angry at this point.*)

THERAPIST: So, I'm not quite clear, but is that what the stress is about?

BETTY: No.

Betty's thoughts seemed to be disconnected from her feelings. I decided on an emotional "perturbation," an interpretation.

THERAPIST: Well, a lot of people in your position might feel pretty angry.

BETTY: (*thinking*) Hmm . . . Maybe! When I talk to my friends about all of this, I notice that I do talk about my supervisor a lot. I basically think I'm upset because I disagree with his way of doing things.

THERAPIST: So does your stress have more to do with how he's doing his job?

BETTY: I think so, and that surprises me . . . I had no idea. . . .

THERAPIST: So if I could wave that magic wand and make it the way you want it to be, what will it be like?

BETTY: I would like to see . . . I wouldn't feel like he's not doing his job. He'd change.

THERAPIST: Do you think you should be able to make that happen?

BETTY: I know I can't really, but . . . I'd feel better.

Betty then gave an example of her supervisor telling her to close her eyes to staff coming in late or taking a long lunch to avoid getting bad evaluations from the staff. Betty was infuriated by this attitude because of its effect on the department's productivity, for which they were responsible above all.

THERAPIST: So what have you tried to do about this?

BETTY: I talk to him, but he always puts off doing anything about it. When I tell him work is running behind he tells me not to worry.

THERAPIST: Well, some people in that situation would be really angry.

BETTY: (looking down in shame and blushing) Ugh . . . nooo . . . angry?

THERAPIST: Don't you think it is OK to be angry in a situation like that? . . . isn't that a normal reaction?

BETTY: Really? Oh, I'm going to cry. (She does.) I think what bothers me most is that I'm acting like this.

THERAPIST: Don't you think a person has the right to be angry sometimes?

BETTY: Oh. That is such a relief.

THERAPIST: You probably aren't used to feeling that way.

BETTY: Not really.

THERAPIST: So, if you were to accept that it is justified to be angry, what could you do about this problem so you wouldn't have to be angry anymore?

Betty began to bite her nails and to look around anxiously while thinking about an answer, so I asked her to recall examples of how she had successfully dealt with problems with her supervisor in the past, other than going over his head. She provided a few examples but the conversation had triggered memories of past fears about complaining and confronting. I became cautious and asked Betty if she wanted to talk about these past fears. She said she did, and I told her to feel free to stop at any time. She shared that when she lost her parents at a young age she was moved from one distant relative's house to another until she grew up. Because she never felt at home anywhere, Betty felt she could never complain or ask for anything no matter how unhappy she was.

When Betty came back a week later she reported that she had had felt in control of her emotions all week. Two weeks later she reported that she feeling like her old self again. She had addressed the need to shore up productivity with her supervisor and he had talked to some staff about punctuality. He had also given her authority to do so. Betty thanked me and said that her goal was reached. She realized that she had issues that she might need to address but she did not want to do that at this time.

Some readers may be disturbed at the idea of terminating this client who clearly could benefit from further work. However, solution-focused therapists are guided by the assumptions that *therapists cannot change clients; clients have to change themselves.* Perhaps this assumption should be rephrased for a situation such as this: *Therapists should not try to change clients; clients must decide when and if they are ready for change.* Moreover, a *small change can lead to bigger changes.* Perhaps when Betty experiences another problem in the future our time together will help her find her own solution; if not, perhaps she will feel comfortable about getting some help. When clients reach the point at which they feel they have achieved what they came for, the solution-focused therapeutic contract is fulfilled. Further sessions can be recommended, but it is up to the client to make the final decision. The exception, of course, would be if there is danger to the client or others, or an unethical situation.

Betty was looking for a solution to being emotionally out of control by searching for a cognitive answer. This was natural for her because she had learned not to allow herself feelings a long time ago. When cooperating with her on that plane did not make a difference for her I cautiously offered a suggestion (perturbation) that her complaint might be anger. This idea resonated with her and helped her find a solution.

Therapy is a collaborative process even if clients can only change as much as they are able to or ready for at a particular time. Offering an emotional suggestion, "Do you think you are angry?," is as valid as a cognitive-behavioral one, "Do you think it would be helpful if you began an exercise program?"

CASE EXAMPLE: NEIL

Neil was a single father who shared child care of his two children, a 7-year-old boy and a 9-year-old girl, with his ex-wife. He made his living as a commercial photographer. He came to therapy because his girlfriend had told him she believed him to be depressed. He knew he had been feeling down for a while but he had not paid attention to it. He admitted that more recently he felt immobilized periodically and even thought about suicide. A suicide assessment indicated that he had considered suicide using pills or cutting his wrists in the bathtub but had such a strong commitment to his children that he did not want them to remember him as having taken his own life.

In the first session he talked mostly about how depressed he was that he might be depressed and could not help himself. When Neil's more open body posture, increased nodding, and better eye contact suggested that he understood that I understood how troubled he felt, I asked how he would know he would not have to come to therapy anymore. He said he would have more energy and more enthusiasm for his relationship and work, but he could not answer whether there were already times when that happened, even in a limited way. I continued to hear Neil describe his distress and to reflect on it. He told me that he had just refused a big project because he did not have the energy to do it. (I see a positive in this negative.)

THERAPIST: That must have been hard to do, but sounds like a good decision.

NEIL: I had to do it. It was the hardest thing to do because I wanted this job badly, but I also didn't want to disappoint the head of the agency. I have worked for him before and he is a great guy. When he sent me the proposal I got so overwhelmed thinking about doing it . . . and it wasn't anything I hadn't done before . . . I just go so overwhelmed, I got nauseated.

THERAPIST: But you had the good sense to take care of yourself! You know your limits.

NEIL: Well, that's not how I thought about it. I hated to do it.

THERAPIST: Was that a different thing for you to do?

NEIL: Well, maybe. . . . I usually push myself as hard as I can.

THERAPIST: Sounds like a wise decision.

NEIL: I felt such relief afterwards.

THERAPIST: I bet. Have you made any other good decisions like that lately? Or taken care of yourself in some good way?

Neil could not think of any examples. He continued to talk about his children and that they were his main motivation in life. He described their weekends together and the fun they had playing board games, making up games of their own, and putting on little plays.

Suddenly Neil stopped and reflected for a few moments. His mood changed and he said:

NEIL: I just remembered something. There was an occasion recently when I felt just a little better and I took care of myself. It was Saturday afternoon. The kids were with their mother . . . I was alone. . . . I decided to just relax and not do any housework. I just sat down and watched TV and didn't worry about anything else I had to do. I even napped a while.

From that point on the conversation moved toward solution. Of course, it is impossible to know what triggered the memory of the exception. One can speculate that because Neil wanted to feel independent and was angry at himself for not being able to help himself, my reflection of some of his behaviors from a more positive perspective changed his perception of himself. That can be considered cognitive reframing. However, it is likely that the context in which reframing occurs, the emotional climate, plays a role in how the reframe is accepted. Notice that it took some time for Neil to respond to our interaction, and I had to keep gauging whether he was ready to talk about a solution. Kiser, Piercy, and Lipchik (1993) pointed out that the movement from problem talk to solution talk should not be considered to happen automatically as a result of the therapist's questions or reflections, because the shift from "affective congruence" (feeling bad and talking about negative experiences) to "affective incongruence" (feeling bad and shifting focus to more positive emotions" (Bower, 1981) often requires time, patience, and clinical skill. I would add that it requires the right emotional climate.

My experience has been that when clients have a difficult time moving away from talking about the problem, allowing some ventilation of feelings, and even intensifying feelings at times, creates a bridge that allows them to face a solution. I was excited to learn that there is actually physiological evidence that thoughts can easily trigger emotions, but it is more difficult to turn off emotions (LeDoux, 1996, p. 303; Panksepp, 1998, p. 301).

During the next six sessions Neil clarified that he had felt terribly angry at himself and helpless because he could not meet all his girlfriend's needs for happiness. As he began to value himself more he recognized that he was not responsible for the relationship alone, and he brought his girlfriend in for couple treatment.

USING OUR OWN EMOTIONS
TO HELP CLIENTS FIND SOLUTIONS

Sometimes clients know what they are feeling and want to talk about it but are afraid, or unable, to do so. This constraint prevents them from finding a solution. Therapists are not mind readers, but we should, as much as possible, be sensitive to clients' nonverbal language as a measure of their emotions. To be as alert as possible to signs of unspoken feelings, we must monitor our own thoughts and feelings. Intuition may be helpful in these situations but should be thought through in an internal conversation before it is offered to clients.

CASE EXAMPLE: SANDRA AND HER DAUGHTERS

Sandra was a 43-year-old, divorced woman who requested a session with her daughters, 16-year-old Rita and 14-year-old Rhoda, as soon as possible. She stated that Rita was moving to another city to live with her father within a week and she needed help in talking with Rita.

The air was heavy and strained when this family came into the room. The sisters looked anxious and spoke in whispers. They said they did not know why their mother had brought them. Sandra, an otherwise pleasant-looking woman, had a mask-like expression on her face and barely moved a muscle as she spoke in a monotone voice. She said she had come because she had had to call the police last week to find Rita, who had always called previously when she was late. When the police brought Rita home, Rita was reported to have been hostile and to have shouted out in front of curious neighbors that she wanted to leave home because she hated the fact that Sandra was a lesbian. The next day Rita asked her mother to make arrangements for her to go live with her father in another city. These plans had now been finalized.

My question about what the family wanted to discuss in the session was met with silence. Sandra expressed pain and disappointment in Rita's behavior. She said the family had never had problems before. She understood if Rita was uncomfortable with her sexual orientation and wanted to live with her father, but she objected to the way Rita was dealing with it. Rita defended herself. Rhoda chose not to take sides and said little.

My own feelings were that Sandra either brought the girls to keep Rita from leaving or to make peace before Rita left. I did not share that because I wanted the family to clarify their own goals.

As the session progressed it became increasingly weighted with problem talk about tensions that had increased in the past months around Rita's dislike for Sandra's partner. I had the feeling that the family needed to refocus on the purpose of having come and did so by tapping into a resource: Sandra's statement that the family had never had problems before.

THERAPIST: So, I understand that things were always really good between you, Sandra, and Rita, until the last few months but you haven't really talked about it. There seems to be a lot of pain and anger now. But I wonder whether you could help me out some—to understand your family a little better. Could you tell me a little about what you think is good about your family—some things you are proud of, maybe.

SANDRA: Rhoda, what do you feel proud of?

RHODA: (*shrugging and taking a long time to answer*) I don't know right now.

THERAPIST: Rita, what about you? As you look back now, what good things will you remember about life with Mom and Rhoda?

RITA: Christmas, and when we all went to Florida together.

THERAPIST: Anything on a day-to-day basis?

RITA: Hugs—I like it when my mom hugs me. I can't hug my dad the way I hug my mom. I can hug her any time of day—and I know she likes that, too. I don't want to compare or anything, but I can't do that with my dad. It feels good. I also like it when she cooks for me.

THERAPIST: How about good things with your sister?

RITA: I'm going to miss going into her room and listening to music with her and swapping clothes.

THERAPIST: You've already given this a lot of thought. I can tell! (*Rita nods assent.*) Did you know that, Mom?

SANDRA: No.

THERAPIST: What good things are you going to miss?

SANDRA: I'm going to miss having two children. . . . (*hesitates for a moment*) We used to go to bowling together, and sing in the church choir. I liked going to school conferences and getting such great reports about Rita all the time. . . . We just got a large-screen TV we enjoy watching and now it will be just Rhoda and I.

When Sandra said, "I'm going to miss having two children," I noticed a physical reaction in myself, like a shock. I sensed Sandra was feeling that Rita's leaving would be like a death, and that she would never see her again. I had an internal conversation to consider whether or not to share this reaction. What could be the disadvantage? Sandra could think I have misunderstood her. The advantage? It could give strong message that I understood the depth of Sandra's desperation. Rita might become more aware of the level of her mother's pain. The benefits of the risk seemed greater than the danger. Given the probability that this might be the only session we had together, I decided to speak.

THERAPIST: You said you will no longer have two children. The way you said it was like . . . like. . . . Of course you won't have two children at home, but it sounded so final. You'll still have two daughters only one will not be in your home. . . . The way you said it, it sounded almost like you were talking about a death rather than a move.

SANDRA: (*sighing deeply*) I guess it has been feeling just like that to me since Rita told me how she actually felt—it feels like a death—it doesn't feel like she's leaving on a visit or just for a year or two. It was so different when my son left home.

THERAPIST: How was it different?

SANDRA: The circumstances were different. He finished high school and was going away to college. We had our difficulties but had reconciled them. I get the feeling that Rita doesn't want to reconcile . . . just to go and forget. And that seems very final to me.

THERAPIST: Is your mother's impression correct? Were you not intending to have a relationship with her in the future?

RITA: No.

THERAPIST: Why do you think she thinks that?

RITA: Probably because we haven't been communicating in a while. She just doesn't know how I feel.

THERAPIST: So what is your idea about staying connected with Mom and Rhoda after you leave?

Rita then began to talk about her hope for continuing contact by telephone and letters with her mother and sister and of holiday visits. She apologized to her mother for having been so indiscreet in front of the police and neighbors. Mother and daughter left reconciled. Sandra later called to thank me and to tell me that she had come to accept that it was a good decision for Rita to live with her father for the time being, and she no longer felt that their relationship was severed.

EMOTIONS AND THE SUMMATION MESSAGE

The "yes set" (Erickson, Rossi, & Rossi, 1976; Erickson & Rossi, 1979) established during the interview and the break and the compliments given at the beginning of the intervention message were considered hypnotic suggestions that lead to a state of relaxation (see Chapter 6). Emotions were never mentioned in connection with this process. However, the understanding and positives conveyed by the summation message to clients who usually expect the therapist to say things are worse than they expect affords a great deal of emotional relief. The resulting relaxation is essential for reasoning and for making the behavioral decisions (Damasio, 1994) necessary for solutions.

CONCLUSION

Elevating emotions to an equal position with cognition and behavior in SFT may seem like a radical step. Yet, if we accept that language and emotion are inseparable how can we exclude emotion from our practice of therapy?

Emotions can facilitate solutions by offering an important way of connecting with and understanding clients (King, 1998). Primary emotions are a universal way of communicating. They occur without conscious control and dependence on words. Infants do not need words to communicate surprise, hurt, or hunger. There is an unspoken emotional connection between clients and therapists in the room that is not transmitted to the therapists behind the mirror. Although we usually converse with clients on the level of emotions that have been refined by physical and mental maturation and socialization, drawing their attention to what Steve Gilligan (1997) calls "an indestructible 'tender soft spot' . . . at the core of each person" can facilitate solutions. One way to do that is to create an emotional climate that provides security (Sullivan, 1956). Another way is to use our own intuition and feelings to help clients become aware of their feelings so they can use them, as well as their reasoning, to find solutions. Of course, it goes the other way as well. Clients who feel only emotion must be helped to access their ability to reason. Clients whose behavior is out of control must be helped to feel and reason. We cannot live productive lives without emotion, and therefore emotion has to be included in solutions for better living.

5

The Process of Clarifying Goals

Some years ago I always used to ask one of these questions in the first session: "How will you know that coming here is useful?," or "If you were to come back next week and tell me that you have noticed a small change for the better, what would that be?" I chose these questions to focus clients on goals. Their answers would inform them and me where they wanted to go. I also believed these questions steered clients away from problem talk. The responses to the questions varied. However, they led to quick solutions only on rare occasions.

About 10 years ago, I stopped using these introductory questions because of what I learned from a workshop I had conducted. The participants had been interviewing each other in small groups and one man shared afterward that he felt angry when his "therapist" asked him the first of the two aforementioned questions. He said he had wanted to tell his story, and the question prevented him from doing so. The subsequent group discussion made me aware that these future-focused opening questions set the stage for therapy by depriving the client of choice. This is not good SFT. The issue should not be when goals are defined but that they reflect as closely as possible what clients want from therapy.

In this chapter I discuss goal clarification as an ongoing process, as opposed to the generally held view that concrete goals should be defined in behavioral terms in the first session if at all possible (Berg & Miller, 1992; de Shazer, 1985, 1991a; Durrant, 1993; O'Hanlon & Weiner-Davis, 1989; Walter & Peller, 1992). The ideas presented apply only for self-referred clients. Chapter 10 discusses involuntary clients.

GOALS VERSUS SOLUTIONS

In keeping with the assumption that *problems don't necessarily have anything to do with solutions,* it follows that neither are problems necessarily related to goals. Clients usually come to therapy with a goal in mind, but that goal may not be the solution. The solution will be whatever clients perceive as making their situation less problematic, or nonproblematic, at a particular time.

Goals are usually conceived in either–or terms; that is, the problem is "all bad" and the solution is "all good." "I will never be angry again," or "We will always be a happy family" are usual but unrealistic goal expectations. These singular thoughts are also poor premises for good mental health and may seem difficult to achieve when all it may take to find a fitting solution is a relatively small change, the difference between two shades of gray.

Solutions are the end product of a process of discovery. They may be far removed from what clients thought their goal was when they entered therapy. Based on this reasoning, "goal clarification" is better thought of as an ongoing monitoring of, and reevaluation with, clients during therapy of what they want the outcome to be. More recently, Walter and Peller (1996, p. 18) described it as a process about evolving meaning and refer to it as "goaling."

THE TASK OF CLARIFYING GOALS

The belief that a goal must be defined by the end of the first session is reinforced by managed care companies that demand concrete evidence that therapists are using their time in a constructive manner. This concept is also useful for quality assurance and research. Indeed, helping clients define what they want from therapy is essential, particularly for an approach as pragmatic and focused as SFT. However, this task must not be taken too literally lest it become the therapist's goal in place of what the client may need at the time. The rush to define goals can put undue pressure on therapists and clients and result in poorly defined goals that lead to dead-end conversations. Moreover, it can be detrimental to the emotion climate of the therapist–client relationship.

The term "goal definition" suggests linearity, precision, and a cognitive process. It implies structure, like a protocol. Some clients are capable of defining a clear behavioral goal at the beginning of therapy that remains consistent. Many others are too overwhelmed emotionally to do any more than articulate some "complaints" (de Shazer, 1985, pp. 31–32). These complaints are usually more vague or general than what is eventually defined as the problem. More often than not, complaints are redefined during the therapeutic process until the client is clear about what the problem is. A clear understanding of the problem usually illuminates the goal or the solution.

CLARIFYING GOALS: THE PROCESS

It takes time and patience to help clients understand what they want from therapy. The assumption that *brief therapy goes slowly* reminds us of that. It helps maintain a flexible attitude, to hear what is being said without listening with intent, and to clarify and ask for meanings only when necessary.

Imagine this scenario: You need a new garment to wear to work or for a particular occasion. You consider your options and make choices about style and color. For example, if you are a woman, you may decide on a red dress. You go to the store and look for an item that fits that description. The first one you find suits you and you buy it. This is possible but unlikely, particularly for a woman. Most people try on several garments that might fit their needs and if they are lucky they will find one they like. More often, while searching through the racks in the store they may be drawn to another color or style of garment than the one they thought they wanted. The woman who thought she wanted the red dress may end up deciding that a black pants suit is more becoming and versatile. The experience of shopping offers options that formulated expectations cannot.

This process is similar to the one our clients go through. Their imagined goals may change when they are offered a chance to think them through from various perspectives. The interaction with the therapist should offer the opportunity to do that.

"Clarifying goals" is a process that begins in the first session and continues until termination. It calls for constant monitoring of clients to make certain we are on the same track as they are (Walter & Peller, 1994). There are questions that suggest themselves automatically for this process, regardless of the stage of therapy:

1. "What do you think the problem is (now)?"
2. "How will you know the problem is solved?"

3. "How will you know you don't have to come here anymore? What will the signs be?"
4. "What will have to be different for that to happen in terms of your behaviors, thoughts, and feelings?"
5. "What will you notice that is different about others involved in the situation?"
6. "What is your wildest fantasy about what you want to have happen?" (Any version of the miracle question serves well for clarification.)

Once there is agreement about the direction, scaling questions can be used to monitor progress toward solution.

The reason it is so important in SFT to help clients clarify their goals is that unless clients are clear about what they really want, they will not be able to recognize a solution. Because *every client is unique,* and *therapists cannot change clients; clients have to change themselves,* only the clients can know when that time has come.

For example, at the beginning of the session a couple may say their goal is to have a more active sex life. Building a solution based on this goal without talking about the context in which that sexual relationship takes place may work if the couple is ready for more intimacy. However, given the assumption that *SFT goes slowly,* it is worth taking the time to explore the context of their sexual relationship first. This exploration may bring forth additional information—for example, a lack of trust about being loved. If the clients would revise their goal and work on increased trust, they might have a better chance for a successful solution than if they continued to work toward a more active sex life, because small steps toward trust represent a lot less risk than steps toward sexual intimacy. Increased trust would probably lead to a more active sex life anyway. Paradoxically, the seemingly less direct route to the solution may result in a quicker solution. The role of the solution-focused therapist is to facilitate the process of self-awareness for clients so that the perturbations will have a greatest probability of becoming fitting solutions for them.

GOALS AND EMOTIONS

Because emotions are part of language, they should be included in clarifying goals. For example, Jonathan described his reason for coming to therapy as "I want to be more decisive." He clarified this reason behaviorally as "I will not question my opinions and choices as soon as anyone challenges them but act on my own decisions." The therapist reflected the emotional side of that description, "So, are you saying you will not be afraid to make your own decisions?" Jonathan's face lit up. "Yes, exactly, that's it!" Now given that Jonathan is a person who likes to please, the therapist had to be careful that Jonathan did not respond positively to the emotional reflection because it came from the therapist. She had to ask Jonathan to make a decision about how he wanted to phrase his goal. Should it be about acting decisively or about not being afraid? They are obviously connected, but Jonathan had to clarify for himself what seemed to be the best description for him. In this case, the request to clarify was also good practice for his decision making as well as increasing the probability of a smooth road to a solution.

Talking about "clarifying goals" rather than "redefining goals" can also have a favorable impact on clients who are not experiencing progress. It is far less jarring for clients to suggest that what they want from therapy has changed and to be asked, "What fits better for you now?," or "What would you prefer to focus on now?," than to imply that a change must occur. Change can be interpreted by clients to mean they set a wrong goal earlier. The feeling that they made a mistake can lead to feelings of shame that disturb the emotional climate.

Some clients are afraid of change, even though they come to therapy for it. This fear is usually manifested by lack of progress, a perception of no progress when some change has occurred, or a relapse. Clients who are ambivalent about change tend to indicate it by directly, or indirectly, expressing negative feelings about themselves, the therapist, or therapy. Once again, given their emotional state, it is far safer to explore their present state of mind about what they want from therapy than to talk about redefining goals. Even a gentle probe, such as "I was wondering whether it would be helpful to check out the goals you defined earlier?," is not worth the risk of evoking shame in clients. Clarifying as part of ongoing conversation provides more security.

CASE EXAMPLE: MARILYN

The following five-session course of treatment over a period of 3 months illustrates my point about clarifying goals as a process instead of a task. It also highlights a therapist's choices discussed in the previous chapters.[1]

---

[1]A version of this case emphasizing a different point was previously published in Lipchik (1993). Copyright 1993 by The Guilford Press. Reprinted by permission.

Marilyn was 30 years old, white, married with a 19-month-old child. She worked part time in a bank. She was a pleasant-looking woman who we might describe as on the upper limit of the weight charts for her height but not yet overweight. Five years ago, right after she was married, Marilyn was seen for six sessions to help her deal with her relationship with her father. This loving but controlling man had had a difficult time sharing his only child with her new husband and was making unreasonable demands on them for time and attention. The solution Marilyn found was to choose how to give him attention rather than to avoid giving him any attention at all.

Marilyn said her goal for coming back to therapy was to "cure an eating disorder." In the process of catching up on the past 5 years, she reported that she was proud that things have continued to go well with her father. She had stopped trying to change him and accepted him as he was. "He still makes comments here and there that I just let fly," she said.

Marilyn described her present problem as follows in an anxious, pressured manner:

MARILYN: I've had a weight problem all my life and I am losing control more and more, you know, and putting on more and more weight, and I just feel like there is some reason that I can't control that . . . my eating habits.

THERAPIST: Was there a time when you could?

MARILYN: When I belonged to Weight Watchers. At that time I lost 30 pounds, but gradually I just went back to the old habits . . . and . . . you know . . . I don't know . . . my goals aren't to have the amount of weight loss I achieved at that time. You know, at Weight Watchers they make you weigh and measure everything. Eating two teaspoons of margarine instead of one is not my problem. That's not what I want to do. *It's the bingeing that's the problem.* [This was the first of Marilyn's statements about what she wanted.]

THERAPIST: Right . . . right . . . so how often do you binge?

MARILYN: Daily.

THERAPIST: What exactly does that mean?

MARILYN: It means I go through the cabinets and the refrigerator and eat anything I find. If I don't find anything, I go to the basement, where we stock things, to find crackers or something.

THERAPIST: [Here I asked Marilyn what this behavior meant to her to promote self-awareness.] How do you explain this to yourself?

MARILYN: It's a long-term thing. Ever since grade school or early high school.

THERAPIST: Oh, really. And daily?

MARILYN: Once in a while when I go on a diet . . . for a while . . . it stops, but generally yes. I try to analyze it, and it's just . . . I don't know . . . it's not necessarily when I'm depressed. I can't associate it with one emotion or another. I just can't explain it.

THERAPIST: It's probably a habit by now. [I picked up on a word Marilyn had used several times.]

MARILYN: Yeah, and it's so irrational. And while I'm eating like that I think, "This is ridiculous," and then I start getting depressed.

THERAPIST: So the only time you don't do that is when you decide to go on a diet?

MARILYN: Yes. When I was on Weight Watchers that was the longest time, probably four months, but then I go back into it gradually. But now it's worse than ever.

THERAPIST: What does Jim think? [Expanding the context of Marilyn's view]

MARILYN: He . . . you know, I cry and say I have to get control . . . and when I join Weight Watchers he thinks it's a good idea, but then he's had this attitude all along that I'm not going to maintain this way of eating. I like all the fatty foods. I never stick to it.

Marilyn went on to describe that she started looking for food as soon as her husband left for work and then ate for about an hour. Did she think it had anything to do with his leaving? She did not. What did she eat? She liked lunchmeats such as bologna and liverwurst, crackers of all kinds, junk food, and peanut butter, which she ate out of the jar like ice cream. Lately, she found herself eating cold leftovers from the refrigerator after eating her regular dinner.

Marilyn described always eating in front of the TV in the kitchen. When she was busy she ate less, but she often found herself feeling "too lazy" to keep busy and stayed in front of the TV. When she noticed that she was being lazy she got angry at herself and started to eat. Weekends were reported to be better, although Marilyn said she would binge even then, when her husband was out of the house. "I don't eat like that in front of anyone, even Jim," she said. Expanding on "being busy" did not lead anywhere.

My internal conversation on my dual track was registering Marilyn's process. She talked about wanting change but rejected all possibilities for it. The old "yes, but" routine! She continued to express anger at herself. I sensed discomfort and realized that I felt that the conversation was becoming too negative, so I asked a miracle question to focus on a different future.

MARILYN: If a miracle happened I'd probably eat a little bit of chips . . . junk food, popcorn . . . I'd definitely not eat leftovers. That's like eating another dinner. I'd have some control.

THERAPIST: What percent of the time would you say you are out of control?

MARILYN: Ninety percent.

THERAPIST: How much control do you think you will have to gain to feel comfortable?

MARILYN: At least 75 to 80% in control.

THERAPIST: OK . . . and . . . well, that is not going to happen right away. Ninety percent out of control to 75% in control . . . big leap. How will you begin to see a 5% change? What will that look like to you?

MARILYN: Either stop sooner and have 1 or 2 days when I'm not . . . let's say 5 days, 10 binges, eliminate 1 or 2 or 5% . . . something like that.

THERAPIST: Which do you think is easier for you? Stopping sooner or eliminating some? [This broadened choices from either–or to both–and, and relieved some emotional tension from the struggle between the two.]

MARILYN: Probably eliminating one, or at least change it to a snack, instead of a binge . . . allowing myself something but not allowing myself to be out of control.

THERAPIST: So when you choose a time and what to eat, when that happens, what do you imagine you will have to do to stick to that and not feel dissatisfied?

MARILYN: Probably do something.

THERAPIST: Like?

We returned to exploring Marilyn's idea of "doing something" instead of eating, but she diverted to deprecating herself again. The people with whom she worked are all slim and diet conscious and she was afraid they all thought of her as a person who lacked control.

It was becoming clear Marilyn was not ready to work on a solution. On the other hand, I wanted to avoid further self-deprecation, so I asked an advantage question. I could have gone back to pursuing the miracle question but chose an advantage question instead. The purpose of the advantage question is to stimulate some both–and thinking because it asks clients to consider what is positive about the negative.

THERAPIST: I know this question may sound strange to you. I want you to realize I am hearing your stress and concern, but what would you say is the advantage of having this problem?

MARILYN: That's a good question. Well, I am finding that I don't go up to people I know, say in a restaurant. Maybe I use it as an excuse to do that. I don't know.

THERAPIST: Why would you want to avoid that?

MARILYN: Because I feel fat.

THERAPIST: Anything else?

MARILYN: I can eat as much as I want to and not think about it—that saves a lot of energy.

THERAPIST: How can you have those advantages without having the problem you came in for?

MARILYN: Mm . . . stopping fighting with myself, I guess.

THERAPIST: Fighting with yourself?

MARILYN: Oh, you know, telling myself I should not be eating so much but wanting to anyway.

THERAPIST: Is that what happens when you binge?

MARILYN: *Yes, that's really the problem, being angry at myself for wanting to eat.* [She redefined her problem once again.]

I had heard Marilyn present her problem in many different ways: eating disorder, bingeing, bad habit, being out of control, and being angry at herself. All these seemed to boil down to her getting angrier at herself the less control she felt. Because her solution with her relationship with her father had been one of gaining control, I referred back to this resource.

THERAPIST: What do you think made a different for you when you came to see me after your marriage, about your father?

MARILYN: I remember . . . ugh . . . you asked me what my options were in how to deal with my father, and I had never thought what my options were. One of them was not to have contact with my parents. I did not want that. You made me think of how I wanted to approach this and just asked me questions that gave me ideas.

THERAPIST: What are your options now?

MARILYN: Either accepting things as they are or getting under control.

THERAPIST: What are some of the options between those two? [Both–and]

Marilyn decided that it would be a start if she stopped eating peanut butter out of the jar or ice cream out of the box. But she emphasized again that she did not want to give up the enjoyment of eating, nor did she want a rigid structure around it.

In formulating the summation message and task I considered that it had to address Marilyn's struggle between control and dependence. Therefore, the message reflected my understanding of her control issues while I offered also offered something concrete for her to think about.

THERAPIST: [Summation message] What I heard you say today is that you want to deal with a habit you have had since your high school days . . . fighting with yourself about eating what you want to eat and as much of it as you want to eat, and that it bothers you not only because of how it makes you feel about yourself but also what other people might think about you. You feel that at this time you want individual attention to get control over this problem, not a group program, and that you don't want an eating routine that is very structured and that you won't be able to keep up later. Your husband seems to be giving up on supporting your struggle and is trying to convince you to accept yourself the way you are, as he does.

I also heard you say you have been successful in keeping control of your relationship with your father for the past 5 years and what helped you do that was to think of options.

My response is that your decision now makes a lot of sense because you are a person who when she makes up her mind to do something, does it. If you chose this time to do it, there must be a good reason for it. You have a lot of understanding of what works for you and what doesn't, and because thinking through options worked for you before, that may work for you again.

MARILYN: Maybe I'm unrealistic to want to have it just happen just like that.

THERAPIST: That may be. It may take a little time for you to figure out how you can best stop being angry at yourself and get the right amount of control you want. I am not sure, but maybe it would help to think of options for what type of snacking you want to do, at what times, and what kind of options you have for keeping busy. You might even want to try choosing in the morning how you want to snack, and keep busy that day, and see whether you like that or not.

MARILYN: Good, I'll do that. I just want to reach my prepregnancy weight and get a hold of myself. [I heard that Marilyn now mentioned another possible goal, losing weight, which contradicted what she had said before.]

Second Session (2 Weeks Later)

THERAPIST: So, what happened that you want to continue to have happen?

MARILYN: It was hard, very hard. Sometimes I wonder if it's even possible. I tried all the options religiously the first week, wrote it down, planned it, wrote it down. Then the second week I did it verbally . . . and didn't do so well.

THERAPIST: Tell me about the first week and what worked.

I questioned her in detail about the successful behaviors and learned that she had stopped eating peanut butter and ice cream and had substituted saltines for more fatty crackers. She did not take well to my enthusiasm about these changes and qualified her success by saying, "Well, some days it worked and some days it didn't." I asked "But does that mean that overall you ate less the last 2 weeks than before?" Her reply was "Oh, sure, much less overall, but I also know that I compensate for eating less in one area by overeating in another. Marilyn's reaction to obvious change for the better signaled that she really was not ready for a solution. I had to look to her to try to trigger some motivation in some other way.

THERAPIST: I guess I'm not quite clear at this time what you think would be the most helpful thing to focus on?

MARILYN: Maybe taking it a day at a time. There were a few days when I did not snack at all. [Notice that when I did not challenge her position, she became more positive on her own.]

THERAPIST: What did you do instead?

MARILYN: Well, Ash Wednesday was one day; that gave me a reason.

THERAPIST: What did you do instead?

MARILYN: Oh, I had it all written down, and I found things around the house to do instead. (*angrily*) If I can do it one day or two, why can't I just do it?

THERAPIST: You sound angry at yourself.

MARILYN: I am. *The whole issue is a control issue.* I know other people have the problem too, but look at all my friends. They don't even have to think about it. Why can they and I can't?

I became aware that I was experiencing some frustration with Marilyn's attitude and I remembered that I *cannot change clients; they can only change themselves.* Consequently, I became accepting of Marilyn's position at this moment and just reflected her feelings while she vented more anger at herself. This gradually diminished and the session ended with Marilyn saying that she understood that she must learn to accept herself.

THERAPIST: [Summation message] What I heard you say today is that you realize that your goal for coming here is actually to stop being angry with yourself because of your eating habits . . . and to accept your behavior and what you think others think about it, about controlling your eating, that is. You came in with the expectations to get immediate control. You said your husband said you are OK the way you are and you should accept yourself like he accepts you, but you think if you accept yourself you'll get heavier and heavier.

My response is that you seem to be on the right track by working toward self-acceptance. It is possible that the more you fight yourself the less energy you may have to find options that fit for you. I wonder what you think about changing the way you fight with yourself? For example, one day you make sure you fight all day and the next you don't fight at all and accept yourself.

MARILYN: I don't know how I could stop it for a day.

THERAPIST: But you told me you have done that already at times.

MARILYN: I don't think I could stop the internal argument.

THERAPIST: How did you do it before?

MARILYN: Well, with reasons . . . like Lent or paying Weight Watchers. But I could try this. What should I do?

THERAPIST: On the day you aren't supposed to fight, any time you experience the struggle inside you, tell yourself you have to postpone it for tomorrow because today you can do anything you please. On the alternate days give yourself permission to fight with yourself at every opportunity because the next day you won't be able to.

MARILYN: OK, I'll try that. So what I am working toward is . . . ? I don't know if that part of me would shut off.

THERAPIST: Would you be shutting it off or postponing it?

MARILYN: I think it would work better for me if I did it in small pieces. I think I would allow myself to argue with myself in the afternoon and leave the not arguing toward the end of the day when I am tired, when I have less energy to keep that argument going. [Always allow clients to modify suggestions. They are more likely to do it their way.]

THERAPIST: Any way that you think it will work for you is fine. I just caution you not to expect too much too soon.

Third Session (2 Weeks Later)

Marilyn reported she was doing better in terms of bingeing but actually gained some weight and now wants to work on losing weight. I was surprised at this change but did not comment on it for the sake of the emotional climate. As we continued to talk I became aware that Marilyn was accepting herself more and focusing less on her eating. However, she insisted that the changes were due to the fact that her husband is around a little more and that she had had more things to do, in general. She agreed that she was gaining control gradually but that it was not enough. When Marilyn complained that she had had a lifetime pattern of not maintaining changes and would never be able to maintain control, I reminded her of an important exception: her situation with her father.

In the summation message I compared her struggle with her father to her present one and built the task around her past solution. Marilyn had resolved the former problem by considering her need instead of her father's criticism. I suggested a similar process now: Whenever she noticed that she was being critical of herself she should ask herself whether that was what her father, or others might think about her, or whether that was the way she wanted to think about herself.

Fourth Session (3 Weeks Later)

Marilyn's first comment was that she might have been a little less angry with herself during the preceding 3 weeks. She said she was angry 50% of the time but that was "not good enough." She also reported that she had followed the suggestion I made at the end of the last session and noticed that she felt as though there was a rebellious child inside her. This child was making her eat because it had never been able to get her own way in the past. "It's like the child is saying, 'This is what I really want to do and no one is going to stop me.' " This further clarification of the problem prompted me to ask Marilyn how she, the competent adult, wanted to handle this rebellious child.

MARILYN: *Maybe I should just concentrate on accepting myself.*

THERAPIST: How could you both eat with enjoyment and accept yourself? [Both–and]

MARILYN: I won't have these bad feelings about myself, and I think that the way they seem to come out is through the eating issue.

THERAPIST: Is that the symptom of your feeling bad about yourself?

MARILYN: *It's my worst fault, the thing I'm most mad at myself for.* [She continued to redefine the problem.]

THERAPIST: OK! So if that is what you want to accomplish here, how will you know you are accepting yourself more?

MARILYN: Not having bad feelings about myself again and not hearing "You have no control."

THERAPIST: How did you learn to accept yourself in other situations?

MARILYN: I don't know. There aren't many other areas I don't accept myself in.

THERAPIST: How about as a daughter?

MARILYN: I realized I was not a bad daughter; it wasn't my problem. But this situation is just me.

THERAPIST: So if you were to think of yourself as *both* accepting yourself and critical, like you used to think of your father—how could you respond differently to yourself?

MARILYN: I let him say what he wants to say and I do what I want.

THERAPIST: So how could that translate to being critical of your eating habits?

MARILYN: I guess I'd have to tell that part to shut up.

THERAPIST: That's not how you handle your father.

MARILYN: I ignore him.

THERAPIST: Could you do that to your own criticism?

MARILYN: Yes, I think that's what I have been doing even without realizing when I feel better. I say this is what I choose to do right now.

THERAPIST: Just the week after you come in here or later too?

MARILYN: It's better all the time, although it is much better right after I see you.

THERAPIST: Would you say that as we are working together the percentage of your doing that has increased? How much more accepting are you now than before?

MARILYN: Thirty to 40% more.

THERAPIST: At the beginning you said you were only 10% OK, and now that is 30 to 40% more. That puts it at 50% better.

MARILYN: Now my goal is different though. When I came in it was to lose weight, but not anymore. My clothes didn't fit me, so I went out and bought new clothes. That's a sign of accepting myself.

THERAPIST: It's wonderful that you feel that way. Great!

MARILYN: I know I could lose 10 pounds in 3 weeks if I wanted to, but I just don't want to. So I finally thought, well . . . I'll buy clothes I feel attractive in . . . but then I wonder whether I am just copping out?

THERAPIST: What is your answer to that?

MARILYN: That this is how I am right now. If I can accept myself the way I am now, maybe in a year I'll be lighter . . . or something else will happen. . . . I want to get pregnant. I want to stop thinking of it as though it's either totally good or bad.

THERAPIST: Right now how has that balance changed for you?

MARILYN: My feelings about my eating having changed so that I am much more accepting of my eating habits, but my eating is the same . . . well almost . . . sometimes better, sometimes worse.

THERAPIST: Do you think you could accept making different choices for yourself at different times?

MARILYN: Hm, that's where I'm stuck.

THERAPIST: [Summation message] I heard you saying you are making progress but it is not bringing you results quickly enough. I also heard you say that you are clear now that your main goal is to accept yourself, regardless of your eating habits.

My response is that I think you are on the right track, but the only way to be accepting of yourself is to stop trying to change yourself for a while and to let what happens happen—to stop and see how thing go when you just let go of trying to change yourself . . . maybe for a month or so. Of course, you will still get the critical thoughts sometimes. Some people deal with them by setting aside 10 minutes a day just for that purpose, for thinking all the critical thoughts they have during the rest of the day. Some people find it useful to write down the critical thoughts at that time and then to tear them up and throw them away. I know you don't like to write things down. You might want to find other ways to do that. See what happens!

Fifth Session (5 Weeks Later)

Marilyn reported she was feeling better about everything because she was accepting herself and "looking at the good points as well as the bad." In terms of the eating, she felt more in control. The major change was that she was not fighting with herself as much. "It is such a relief," she said, "just like when I finally stopped fighting with my dad." I asked how this new development affected her daily life and she said that it kept her from getting depressed.

THERAPIST: Is there something similar about having felt out of control in relationship to your father and with food?

MARILYN: I think so. I definitely felt I had no control and he had all. Once I gained control I felt relief.

THERAPIST: Your behavior changed?

MARILYN: Yes, and that stuck.

THERAPIST: Yes, So now you made the same realization about eating and fighting with yourself and being angry at yourself for not having control.

MARILYN: Yes, I don't fight with myself much anymore.

THERAPIST: Really?

MARILYN: Yes

THERAPIST: Two years from now . . . 3 years from now . . . how will this change you made now affect how you will eat in the future?

MARILYN: Hopefully, I won't fight with myself or think about it. I think if I give myself freedom to eat what I want to, I won't eat more. So I cannot see—unless my metabolism changes—that I'll gain a lot more weight than I have now, and I'll be comfortable with that.

At the end of the session I asked Marilyn to scale the difference in her acceptance of herself around eating and she replied that eating was just part of the whole picture and overall she felt 80 to 85% in control as compared to 25% when she first came in. In terms of her confidence that she could maintain these changes she said, "I'm not sure. It's so new."

THERAPIST: And you will have to work on it and keep reinforcing it. One formula for doing that in the future . . . you know it's normal for self-acceptance and self-confidence to go up and down . . . 85% is great now, but it will take time to make it a habit. . . . So, I was thinking, so that you don't feel disappointed if you don't feel at least 85% accepting of yourself . . . when you feel some slippage, think of what you have to do to adjust the balance between self-acceptance and self-judgment rather than letting yourself get torn between all negative or all positive.

Marilyn and I agreed that she had achieved her goal and that we did not have to meet anymore.

The summation message reviewed her goal, her accomplishments and her new way of thinking about this problem.

What is significant about this case is how the process was changing as Marilyn kept clarifying the content. In five sessions she moved from her a goal of "curing an eating disorder" and anger at herself to self-acceptance. The connection on the process level helped her clarify her thinking on the content level.

DECISION-MAKING GOALS

When a client's goal is to make a choice between two or more alternatives we becomes guides in a problem-solving process. We must listen carefully to help the client consider options. Some of the work, such as listing pros and cons, or prioritizing, can be suggested as homework tasks. A variation on this suggestion is to ask clients to list the short- and long-term advantages and disadvantages of their options.

For example, a man comes to decide whether to leave his wife or forgive her for having had a brief affair for which she is remorseful.

The short-term advantage: It saves his pride, and he can hurt her like she hurt him.

The long-term advantage: He will not have to worry about whether he can trust her anymore.

The short-term disadvantage: His whole life will be disrupted and he will lose someone he still has deep feelings for.

The long-term disadvantage: He may miss an opportunity to make some changes in the marriage now that could improve it for the future.

The goal is to make a decision, regardless of what it is. If the client wishes to continue seeing the therapist after that, a new problem will have to be defined based on how the client will know therapy has helped him.

In this particular case, if the man decides to leave his wife the new problem may be how to cope with living as a single person, how to cope with the loss, how to coparent the children, or all of these. If his decision is to forgive and work on the marriage, he and his wife may want marital therapy and will have to define the problem and goals for that together. If the wife does not want therapy and the husband does, the husband will have to define his problem—that is, how to develop trust and/or forgive. On the other hand, the client may leave and not feel the need for further therapy. What he needed from therapy was to make a decision and therefore the contract with the therapist is fulfilled. If he feels satisfied with that as a solution, the therapist must be satisfied as well. It would not fit the solution-focused philosophy to keep the client coming to help him cope with the transition unless the client identified that as a need.

Some clients who come about a decision feel pressured to make it as quickly as possible. Urgency only exacerbates the either–or aspect of decisions. Time to gather and examine necessary information is a better option at that point. Consequently, we should attempt to slow clients down, or help them to postpone the decision for a while, if possible. Suggestions for accomplishing this slowdown is to say we need more time to get to know the situation better, or that it might be better to postpone the decision to be sure it will be the right one.

I recall a case in which a woman came in to make a decision about leaving a boyfriend. He was a 7 on a scale of 10 overall, but she described him as putting his children from his first marriage ahead of her needs. She was anxious to make a decision because she was exhausted from trying to figure out what to do. I wondered whether she would be willing to put the decision on hold for a few weeks while I helped her explore it in greater depth. She seemed to relax and be relieved. I then suggested that because she did not have to make a decision right away she might want to notice what she enjoyed about being with him when he initiated a date. In the next session she reported that she had felt more relaxed that week. Two weeks later she reported that her boyfriend had suddenly become more attuned to her needs and was asking to see her more. She canceled a next session and said that things were going so well and she had decided to remain in the relationship.

Another useful question to ask clients when they are uncertain about making a decision is, "What do you have to do now (or decide to do now) so when you remember it (or look back at it) in the future you will feel good about yourself?" This question is often much more effective than a miracle question because some people are unable to imagine a better future but everyone is able to remember having made a poor decision and how it made them feel afterward.

THE CLIENT WHOSE GOAL IS
TO CHANGE SOMEONE ELSE'S BEHAVIOR

Successful solutions require clients to take responsibility for their behavior. However, some clients are convinced that their problem would disappear if someone else's behavior changed. The typical example is the parent who wants the therapist to "fix" his or her child or partner.

This type of case, like others, calls for cooperating with the client first of all.

Marjorie came to talk about her unhappiness in her marriage of 15 years to Fred, whom she described as selfish, dishonest, and irresponsible about money. Marjorie and Fred both worked hard and earned about the same income, but while Marjorie deprived herself of many things she would like to buy, Fred indulged himself by buying electronic toys, which wrecked their budget. Marjorie had tried to deal with this problem by insisting that Fred hand over his paycheck and ask her for spending money. This solution appeared to work for a while but Marjorie now felt that Fred had become increasingly uncooperative and tried to sabotage her plans. He had also stopped fulfilling his responsibilities, such as having their car serviced and cutting the lawn. Recently Marjorie planned an anniversary party for her parents and Fred drank too much and belittled her in front of everyone. Marjorie asked Fred to come to therapy with her but he refused.

Clients, too, have to understand that therapists *can't change clients; clients have to change themselves.* When the therapist asked Marjorie how she would know she wouldn't have to come to therapy anymore, she answered that Fred's behavior would have changed. Was Marjorie willing to do something different to make that happen? The answer was, "Absolutely not." Marjorie said there was nothing a therapist could suggest that she had not tried herself. She had tried asking politely that Fred stay within their budget; she had had temper tantrums; she had asked Fred's mother to talk with him about their situation; she had tried talking when he was in a mellow, romantic mood; she had tried refusing to be intimate with him. Nothing had made a difference. She wanted professional help. The therapist first tried to help the client redefine the problem and do something different herself. She wondered whether Fred had ever made changes in his life before, either in relation to her or to others. Marjorie had to think about that a while and then said she thought he changed being late to work because he was threatened with being fired. Did Marjorie think Fred would change if he believed she would leave him? Marjorie instantly replied that she would never leave Fred. It was against her religious conviction and even if it were not, Wisconsin has a joint-property divorce law and she did not want to divide their accumulated assets.

What are the options when we are presented with a situation such as this one? The most therapeutic thing to do is to be honest and tell the client that we cannot change other people. All we can realistically offer is an exploration of options. One option might be how to cope better with the situation. Marjorie was not satisfied with this answer and chose to terminate. However, that is not to say that the therapist's position did not serve as an intervention. Some clients decide to do something else on their own when therapists declare themselves helpless.

CONCLUSION

On the surface, talking about "clarifying goals" rather than "goal definition" seems picayune. What is so different about asking questions as part of a process rather than as a task? The difference is mainly in the implication, which in turn affects the therapist–client interaction. Thinking "process" rather than "task" implies a flow that keeps our mind open to other possibilities. It keeps tweaking our curiosity about where the client is rather than assuming that he or she is at a place determined earlier. The belief that the goal is "set" can restrain and lead to impasse.

At every turn in SFT, we must look to our clients to decide what their goals for therapy are. Not only are they the only ones who can know precisely how they will know that they no longer have to come to therapy, but only they can be the source of their ability and readiness to reach that point. Therefore, it will benefit us to remain patient, flexible, and curious (Cecchin, 1987) throughout the process.

The issue of what clients want and whether they are ready to achieve it is an important part of formulating the summation message and tasks that are discussed in Chapter 7.

6

The Team Behind the Mirror and the Consultation Break

"Teams of observers are most commonly used by structural, Milan, and strategic therapists" (Nichols & Schwartz, 1995, p. 521). Probably the best description of their function comes from the Milan team itself (Selvini Palazzoli et al., 1978, p. 16):

> We all feel that continual supervision by the two colleagues in the observation room is indispensable. External as they are to what occurs in the treatment room, they are less easily drawn into the play and can observe in perspective in a global manner as it were, as if they were spectators watching a football match from the grandstands. The fame on the field is always better grasped by the observers than by the protagonists themselves.
> —SELVINI PALAZZOLI ET AL., 1978, p. 16)

More recently, Tom Andersen (1991, 1995) introduced a more collaborative variation on the team concept, the "reflecting team." In this process clients observe the team discussion behind the mirror and later comment on it.

Originally, the observers behind the one-way mirror at the Brief Family Therapy Center acted as detached observers who never directly communicated with the clients. They assisted the interviewing therapist in composing a message for the client, during a break at the end of the session, but they did not include themselves in that message. Clients were told of the presence of observers behind the mirror, but the observers were purposely not identified. We believed that there was some benefit to an aura of mystery. That changed when a client once asked for feedback from the observers (Nunnally, de Shazer, Lipchik, & Berg, 1986) and the resulting interchange made us realize that the direct connection between clients and the team adds another dimension to the process. Observers now began to make calls from behind the mirror to the therapist, or directly to clients, sometimes to ask questions and other times to comment. These questions and comments from observers could often be used to challenge clients in a way that an interviewing therapist could not do without endangering the relationship. As it happens, Selvini Palazzoli and her group (1978) in Milan and a group at the Ackerman Institute in New York (Papp, 1980) were using the team in the same manner.

The therapist in the room and the observers behind the mirror have different experiences of the interview. These varying impressions provide a richer source of information for intervention message that can also shorten treatment. Unfortunately, most private practitioners in the United States today do not have the luxury of time, or the availability of staff, to do teamwork regularly, if at all. The majority of teamwork is done at universities and training institutes for educational purposes and research.

BENEFITS FOR THE THERAPIST

Teamwork and a break toward the end of the session are powerful ways to help clients. Such collaboration is intellectually and emotionally supportive for the therapists and can prevent burnout. However, the break is valuable in itself, even without a team. Those of us who are accustomed to taking breaks to formulate a closing message and task for clients usually have stories to tell about the occasions we decided to forgo the break to save time. Instead, we may just pause, collect our thoughts quickly, and offer some feedback and a task. Later that afternoon, perhaps on our way home at night, when we reviewed our day, it suddenly became clear that we failed to see the obvious and what we missed telling the clients. Fortunately, there is a way to correct such a situation, although it takes some extra work. A letter to the client sharing the afterthought has the advantage of permanency. It can be read and reread. It is also good for the relationship because it suggests to clients that their therapist is thinking about them even when they are not in his or her presence.

Formulating a message and task while being emotionally and cognitively engaged in a conversation with a client is difficult. Such a feat requires reviewing what the client thinks his or her problem and goals are, what else the client said in this and past sessions, and what our reactions to it are. Of course, there are times when this can be done successfully, but such times usually occur toward the end of therapy, when things are going well and all one needs to say is "keep doing what you are doing." Teamwork can accomplish this task more effectively.

When a team is not available, the best substitute is to take a break by ourselves. The change of environment from the interviewing room to another location moves the therapist from "doing" to "reviewing." These are two different experiences which, when added together, provide more than the sum of its parts for understanding our clients, our interactions with them, and how to respond to them.

BENEFITS FOR THE CLIENTS

The benefits of teamwork and the consultation break for clients are obvious. They offer clients "more then one head working for them" as well as quality assurance. According to Erickson's five steps of trance induction (Schmidt & Trenkle, 1985, p. 143), the process of waiting while the therapist is on a break and then hearing what the team has to offer benefits clients in the following manner:

1. It heightens attention on what the therapist will say upon his or her return.
2. It leads to relaxation when the therapist's message expresses acceptance and understanding.
3. It offers difference by means of surprise, relief, and distraction from client's view of the problem.
4. It offers continuity because it reflects the client's language and manner of cooperating.
5. In a trance-like state, clients are more receptive to information.

Clients usually respond to this process by nodding their heads or smiling with recognition. This response is referred to as a sign of a "yes set" (de Shazer, 1982; Erickson & Rossi, 1979; Erickson et al., 1976), or that the clients are in a state of attentiveness and agreement.

INTRODUCING THE TEAM AND THE BREAK

Most people think of therapy as a private event. They expect a setting in which they will feel free to air their problems and emotions safely. The team approach calls for the use of a one-way mirror or a video hook-up that allows for observation of sessions. This exposure is threatening to some clients and takes sensitivity and skill to sell. Probably the most decisive factor for getting clients to agree to the team approach is how it is presented. The presentation should never be done in a hesitant or apologetic manner. It should reflect pride about the opportunity to give clients such special care. When we believe in this procedure, clients rarely object to it. For example:

"We practice in this manner to be most helpful to you,"
or
"You get more help because several heads are better than one,"
or
"We find we can help more quickly this way,"
or all of these.

Students who are uncomfortable being observed themselves often have a difficult time getting permission for team observation because they project their own discomfort. The more comfortable the therapist is with the process, the more comfortable clients are with it. Sometimes, clients say that they do not mind being observed as long as the observers are in the same room during the interview. Although this defeats the purpose to some extent, it is better to agree to it because it still offers different perspectives and it preserves the emotional climate.

Some other options for getting permission for the team approach are as follows:

1. Explain the team approach to clients on the telephone before they come to the first session.
2. Provide clients a written description of the team approach at intake, before entering the therapy room. This should be reviewed again after clients enter the therapy room.
3. Introduce clients to team members with an invitation to ask them any questions they want to ask.

My own opinion is that clients should have the right to make a decision about team observation. However, it depends on the policy of the particular agency and team whether the client's decision is honored or whether the client is referred elsewhere if he or she refuses. It may be a somewhat more controversial issue in private practice, where most clients come by choice. Although there should not be different standards for people who are mandated to treatment, the reality is that they usually have fewer choices. Thus, the "no other option" alternative is likely to cause the client who receives free or government-subsidized care at a not-for-profit agency to be more agreeable than a private client. This may also be true for anyone seeking treatment at a hospital or university clinic where the team approach is part of a teaching protocol. The important thing to remember under all circumstances is to invite clients to discuss their reluctance and to be patient about explaining the benefits of teamwork.

PRAGMATICS OF TEAMWORK AND THE BREAK

Many therapists work in settings in which it is not practical to take a break. They may be working in an agency that lacks the necessary space. In-home therapists may find it awkward to ask clients to use another part of their home, or to ask that they leave the room for a while. The next best option is to put the message and task into a letter and send it to the client right after the session.

Another consideration is time. Today, more than ever, therapists are under the gun to see as many clients as possible. That mandate often makes it difficult for them to take a break. They need 10 minutes between their sessions to write progress notes or to refresh their memories about the next client. They are reluctant to shorten a 45- or 50-minute session to 35 minutes, to make time for the break and to read the message. I would urge those therapists who feel uncomfortable about shortening their sessions to reconsider. The benefits clients get from a carefully designed summation message and task may well outweigh the extra 10 minutes of conversation.

The break, unlike team observation, should not be offered as a choice. It should be introduced at the beginning of treatment, in a routine, professional manner as information about what the client can expect from therapy. Clients usually respond favorably because the break suggests that they will be getting thoughtful attention.

Following is an example of how to introduce the break:

"I want to let you know that I will be taking a short break toward the end of the session to think over what we talked about today

. . . so that I can sum it up for you and tell you what I'm thinking, or what I might suggest."

TEAM PROCESS

A team can consist of one or more observers. A group of five or less, including the interviewing therapist, is most manageable. Too large a group can produce too much input for a concise message in the allotted time. The solution-focused team's function is to observe the interview and participate in it via phone connection or other means, to participate in a discussion during the break behind the mirror, and to compose a message for the family.

The Milan team took as much time as it needed to formulate an intervention message (Tomm, 1984, p. 255), but most therapists who practice in the United States today are confined to 45- to 60-minute sessions. A practical time frame to consider is 35 minutes for the interview, 10 minutes for the break, and the rest of the time to present the message and get reactions to it from the clients. Those who have the luxury of taking more time when they see a family will appreciate the benefits of not having to work under such tight time constraints.

THE DUAL PERSPECTIVE OF CLIENTS

The face-to-face experience with clients and from behind the mirror differs greatly. Anyone who has had the opportunity to become the interviewing therapist after having been a team member will attest to that. It is not uncommon that any irreverent and judgmental thoughts we had behind the mirror fade on face-to-face contact. This experience suggests that some nonverbal aspects of clients' language that allow for connection, perhaps on an emotional level, are screened out behind the mirror. The view from behind the mirror has the advantage of permitting more spontaneous reaction than an interviewing therapist can allow him- or herself, and also permits a more detached assessment of process, particularly between the clients and the interviewing therapist. The combination of the two perspectives, however, is ideal, and impossible for a therapist to attain without a team.

Imagine a therapist and a team working with a couple that reports incessant fighting. The interviewing therapist cooperates with them by exploring content with them, the details about their fighting. As they move from one issue to another the wife take some responsibility for her part in the fights and her body language conveys openness, while the husband blames the wife for it in a cavalier manner and his nonverbal stance appears evasive. The team behind the mirror wonders about the process and phones in a question asking the couple to rate their commitment to the relationship on a scale from 1 to 10. The answers to the scaling questions will shift the focus of the conversation from content to the deeper issue of their commitment to the relationship. Thus the view from behind the mirror that can assess content and process from a more detached position can facilitate the progress of therapy.

To be helpful, the team must remain aware of its process in relation to the clients' process. I recall a case in which a couple came in because they were unable to make a decision about which of two cities to live in. During the break the team broke into two camps that argued with each other about which task to assign, until one team member pointed out the parallel between the clients' and the team's process.

Once this team recognized that it was caught in the couple's either–or process it formulated the following message for the couple:

"We understand that you each want your own way, but you also want it to please your partner—that is a difficult position to be in. We suggest you go home and think about which is more important, the relationship or getting your own way? Notice if your answer opens up new ideas for solutions."

TEAMWORK AND THE EMOTIONAL CLIMATE

If it is important that the relationship between therapist and clients takes place in the context of a secure emotional climate, it follows that this is also true for the relationship of team members with each other (be they colleagues or supervisor and trainees, and with the clients (Cantwell & Holmes, 1995). Therefore, it is important for team members behind the mirror to be accepting of each other's opinions as well as the interviewing therapist's conversation with clients. Suggestions for the interviewing therapist are best communicated with the same respect and sensitivity that is extended to clients. A favorable emotional climate among therapists will facilitate treatment just as conflict among team members will undermine it.

Calls from the team into the interviewing room should be considered carefully and limited to the most salient ones so as not to disrupt the interview too much. Interruptions are useful but can be disturbing to clients as well as to therapists. It is best for one person behind the mirror to relay questions or comments. These messages should be as clear and short as possible to avoid confusing the interviewing therapist.

Larger teams generally assign one member to speak with the therapist during the break. Other team members offer their information to the designated speakers during the session, or after it, in writing.

Whether the interviewing therapist is to repeat a question called in verbatim or has the liberty to rephrase it must be discussed beforehand and may vary depending on the expertise of the therapeutic team. Generally, it is more useful to ask the interviewing therapist to repeat the question as it was asked, if he or she is a trainee. Calls among experienced therapists may be more of a miniconsultation and take the form of a question such as "I notice you are persisting to stick with the content. Is that deliberate or do you want to consider addressing the power struggle?"

When interviewing therapists join the team behind the mirror, they are always allowed to give their impressions first. The opinion of the person who was in the emotional field with the clients during the interview is generally considered to have a little more weight than that of observers behind a mirror. Breunlin and Cade (1981) suggest that

> the interviewing therapist decides when he has enough information and whether he wants to write the message in his own language or have direct quotes from team members. The final decision to use an idea or message rests with the therapist because he is the one who must ultimately execute and is the most accurate judge of the affective climate of the session. (p. 456)

When the team approach is the standard procedure for all clients, a decision has to be made beforehand whether the interviewing therapist has the authority to make independent decisions about the case. If clients call the interviewing therapist with a question between sessions, does the interviewing therapist answer it or does he or she have to consult the team before answering? Most teams give the interviewing therapists the authority to answer for practical reasons, as well as the fact that the composition of teams is not always stable. There may also be times at which the interviewing therapist will consult some or all of the team members for therapeutic reasons.

For example, a client may call and say she just discovered her married lover is having an affair with another woman and she is so angry that she wants to call his wife and tell her about his affair with her and the other woman. The client wants the therapist's advice whether or not to do this. A solution-focused therapist cannot, in clear conscience, give a direct answer no matter how much he or she disapproves of an action. His or her task is to help the client explore all the aspects of this action, including the morality of it, but the client has to take the consequences for the decision. Thus, in such a case, the therapist saying he will consult with the team gives the client some more time to consider her actions, and gives the therapist time to formulate a carefully composed message. For example, he can be confrontive without jeopardizing his relationship with the client by saying, "Half the team thinks it is understandable that you are so angry that you want revenge, but you should be sure you won't have any regrets afterwards. The other half of the team thinks 'two wrongs don't make a right'." In general, decisions about how to handle between-session calls should be made with an eye to preserving the emotional climate in the interviewing room.

Chapter 7 is devoted to what I call the "summation message" and the "suggestion."

The Summation Message and the Suggestion

The summation message and the suggestion are closely related, yet their formulation may be based on different information about the client. Therefore, they are treated in separate sections here.

THE SUMMATION MESSAGE

What I call the summation message is generally referred to as the intervention message. My idea about changing it to a summation was prompted by the theoretical shift from problem focus to solution focus. The change from interrupting problem-maintaining behavioral patterns to reinforcing nonproblematic behaviors, thoughts, and feelings made the therapeutic process a much more collaborative and less strategic process than before. The customary structure of the "intervention message" was to provide compliments, a clue, and a task (de Shazer, 1982, pp. 42–46). This seemed incongruous with the cooperative tone of the interview because it sounded like a medical diagnosis and prescription. Consequently, the summation message was designed to make the message at the end of the session reflect the question/response pattern of the interview (see Figure 2, p. 31). It consisted of the following:

1. A response by the therapists/team of what they "heard" or understood about the clients' situation.
2. A question to clients about whether they agreed with this response and an acknowledgement of corrections, if necessary.

3. Another response by the therapists/team that offered new information or a different perspective, including a suggestion.

The success of the summation message most likely depends on
whether our formulation of what we heard and how we respond to it fit
with the clients' way of perceiving their situation. The message is most
likely to fit when it is based on content and uses the clients' language
and metaphors. In the context of the theory described in Chapter 1, the
summation message and the suggestion can be thought of as a perturbation to the clients' inherent organization but never as an intervention
that can produce specific change.

Lily and Tom were another couple that came for help to stop fighting. They professed love for each other and to have a lot of common interests and goals, yet they reported major differences about the management of their finances, their sexual relationship, and their relationship
with Lily's parents (content). The couple chose finances as the first issue
on which to work. As the session proceeded the therapist noticed that
every time either partner expressed an opinion the other disagreed and
looked at the therapist for affirmation (process). In keeping with the idea
that a summation message should be formulated in terms of content but
should address process, the therapist offered the following idea (reframe)
to the couple after telling them what he heard about their reasons for
coming to therapy:

"People often fight a lot not because they want to get their way
but because they are fighting to be acknowledged and affirmed
by the person most important in their life."

The suggestion was also built on this reframe:

"Here is a suggestion you may want to think about until we meet
again. How do you want your husband/wife to show you respect
and love around financial issues and how do you want to show
it to them?"

Solution-focused therapists often worry about formulating the
"right" message. However, there is no way of knowing what the right
message is for a particular client at a particular time. Any one of a number of messages may be equally helpful as long as they fit with how clients see their situation. The best we can ever do in summarizing and de-

veloping a suggestion is to use what we understand the client to have expressed in combination with our theoretical assumptions, our experience as therapists, our general knowledge about human behavior, and our intuition. One way to describe an effective summation message is that it gives a good idea about the content and process of the session to anyone who reads it or hears it, even if he or she was not present at the session.

The Structure of the Summation Message

The summation message begins with a summation of what the therapist heard the client say during the interview, starting with the words: "*What I heard you say* [or tell me] today. . . . " This paragraph includes (in a first session):

1. The stated complaints and/or problem.
2. The historical background to the present situation.
3. The clients' description of what they want to have happen.
4. Presession progress and strengths.
5. Anything clients say about how they feel emotionally.

In subsequent sessions:

1. Clients' reports of what happened since the last session in terms of change.
2. Clients' reactions to change, or no change.
3. Any new information the clients reveal, including strengths, resources, feelings.

The summation message should be delivered in a conversational tone and continue the emotional climate of the interview. Each client in the room, regardless of age, should be personally addressed during both parts of the message.

Case Example: The B Family

"What I heard you tell me today, Mr. and Mrs. B, is that you have come here at the suggestion of the school psychologist. The school reports that Tina does not pay attention in class and doesn't get her work done. It is also reported that Tina is alone a lot at school. The reason for it may be that she gets angry so fast that the children don't want to play with her.

"You told us that this school behavior has been getting worse since she started the first grade, just about the time you, Mr. B, started your own business, and you, Mrs. B, began to work second shift. You mentioned that she became more uncooperative and angry at home around that time, as well. You are very concerned and want to do everything you can to help Tina.

"You have tried a number of things to solve this problem such as consulting with the school and several other therapists. At one point you were instrumental in having Tina moved to another classroom with a more patient teacher, but it did not seem to make a lasting difference. You have also tried reward programs, gymnastic classes, reading books on parenting, and working closely with the school. You told us that in terms of discipline, your philosophies generally differ and you often do not find common ground.

"You have come here today to continue to try to help Tina. Mrs. B, what you want to have happen is that Tina listens to adults more at home and at school. Mr. B, you said what you want to see as a result of coming here is that Tina is happier, overall. You think she will conform more when she feels better about herself.

"Mike, we heard you say that you try to ignore the problems at home. You just want everyone to be happier.

"Tina, you said that you would like things to change for you at school and at home. You'd like to have more friends at school and not have your parents so angry with you all the time.

"Did I hear all of you correctly? Is there anything of importance that I omitted, or that you want to add?"

The first section is followed by a statement reflecting the therapist's reaction to the clients starting with: "My response to what I heard you tell me today is. . . . " This is an important section for reinforcing the emotional climate and for offering clients a different point of view. The information related at this point also leads directly into the suggestion.

In a first session, this section should include (not necessarily in this order) the following:

1. A statement reflecting the therapist's empathy and/or acceptance, such as "I'm not surprised you are so depressed"; "What you

have described sounds like a very painful situation"; "It seems like a good idea that you have come to talk to someone."

2. A reflection about the emotional impact of the situation on the client, whether or not he or she has expressed it. "My sense was that you are really hurting a lot!" "I can understand why you would feel that way."

3. Compliments or positive recognition of presession changes, ideas for future changes, existing strengths, and resources.

4. Difference—normalizations, reframes, information about child development, or relationship dynamics; the therapist's reflections or opinions.

5. In the case of a couple or family a shared feeling or goal, that is, both partners are hurting badly, everyone wants to fight less, everyone wants to live in a happy family.

Case Example (Continued from Above)

"Our response to what you told us is first of all, that we think it is a good idea that you decided to come here today, Mr. and Mrs. B, and that you brought Tina and Mike. You all helped a lot to give us a picture of your situation. We noticed that you all basically seem to want the same thing: for things to be better for everyone in the family—for everyone to feel happier. That says something to us about how you care about each other and your family.

"We were impressed that you, Mom and Dad, agree not to leave a stone unturned to help Tina in spite of your busy lives. You are trying to do everything good parents can do . . . and you also have to attend to your work and the house and aging parents. It's a lot.

"In terms of your different philosophies about discipline, we find that that can sometimes be helpful. All children do not respond well to the same style of discipline. So two heads can sometimes be better than one to decide on a consistent plan [a positive way to reframe their disagreement].

"Mike, we really appreciated your honesty in telling us that you try to ignore the problems at home. Many kids might not have been that honest. You impress us as caring a lot about your whole family and not wanting to add to the problems. You just want everyone to be happier.

"Tina, you should be proud of yourself that you are grown up enough to admit that you want things to change. It's a hard thing to do to admit you have done things wrong. But it's often the first step to making things better for yourself and others. "Do you have any comments or questions?"

You will notice that the summation message reflects and continues the listening/responding pattern of the conversation in the interview. The compliments are woven into the response. There is something respectful about checking with clients whether we have heard them correctly. It also enhances their trust in the therapists/team. When I switched to saying "What I heard you say" instead of starting the message with compliments I experienced the "yes set" response (de Shazer, 1982; Erickson et al., 1976; Erickson & Rossi, 1979) (clients showing agreement by nodding their heads) becoming even more noticeable.

THE SUGGESTION

The decision about what suggestions to give clients at the end of sessions seems to be one of the most perplexing problems for therapists. There have been numerous attempts to provide guidelines (Brown-Standridge, 1989; de Shazer & Molnar, 1984; Fisher, Anderson, & Jones, 1981; Haley, 1976; Molnar & de Shazer, 1987; Papp, 1980; Rohrbaugh, Tennen, Press, & White, 1981; Todd, 1981) centered largely on expectations of client compliance (i.e., direct for motivated and indirect for unmotivated, or behavioral vs. cognitive).

The tasks originally used at the Brief Family Therapy Center were similar to the Mental Research Institute "paradoxical" interventions that strove for indirect, systemic pattern interruption to allow the system to reorganize in its own way (Frankl, 1960; Haley, 1973, 1976; Watzlawick et al., 1974) and the counterparadoxical prescriptions of the Milan team (Selvini Palazzoli et al., 1978). They were all intended to circumvent resistance by coupling positive connotation of a dysfunctional pattern with a prescription to continue it, hoping the client will do the opposite. When Brief Family Therapy became SFT the concept of client "cooperation" replaced resistance (de Shazer, 1984). This made it theoretically impossible to prescribe a paradoxical task, because tasks were now based on how clients cooperated so that they would be accepted. In practice, this can actually look much the same. For example, a client who has a competitive manner of cooperating may be told that a particular task works for some clients but would probably not work for him.

I chose the word "suggestion" instead of "tasks" because it is more in keeping with the solution-focused belief *that clients have the resources to help themselves.* For the same reason, I do not think it benefits clients to be labeled customers (de Shazer, 1988; Fisch et al., 1982), complainants, or visitors (de Shazer, 1988) to determine whether they should be given a task. Customers are said to be people who are motivated to change and are therefore likely to try to do something different. Complainants are people who think there is a problem but are not motivated to do much about it. They may or may not do an assignment and should not be given a direct assignment. They might just be asked to notice something. Visitors are people who do not think there is a problem and who do not want to be there. They are expected not to do assignments because they have no motivation and should therefore not be given any. These labels do not necessarily predict client responses (Fish, 1997). Visitors can become customers, and customers can become complainants as a result of their relationship with the therapist in an initial session and thereafter. Customers have even been known to turn into visitors if they had a negative experience. The emotional climate of the interview and the message at the end of the session can significantly alter the attitude a client came in with. Given all this uncertainty, it seems shortsighted not to make a suggestion for change to everyone present. However, keeping it a suggestion rather than an assignment allows clients the choice of acting on it, adapting it to suit their situation better, or ignoring it. Regardless of their response, the emotional climate will be preserved because they can do no wrong.

Tailoring Suggestions

A listing of the well-known solution-focused suggestions can be found on pages 119–121. However, it must be understood that they, too, require careful consideration in terms of fit. Even the Formula-First Session Task is not an appropriate choice in every case. It is intended to interrupt the clients' focus on negatives, but can one ask someone who is dealing with a significant loss what he or she does not want to change? Or how cooperative is it to ask clients what they do not want to change if they are describing a totally negative situation?

Ultimately, the most effective way to develop suggestions is to tailor them to the individual case. Tailoring suggestions is not as difficult as it may seem, and it can be fun, because it is a creative process. Suggestions are based on logical thinking about information that was generated in the session about who clients are and what they want and using that information to imagine what kind of an experience will make a difference for them. Thus, if we heard about positive change in a session and rein-forced it in the summation message with compliments, we are prompted to think about a suggestion that will keep that positive change going. If we heard that the situation is the same, or worse, we are prompted to think about suggestions that will either prevent things from getting worse or lead to small improvements. A message that reflects how badly a husband and wife are hurting because they both feel unappreciated prompts us to come up with ideas that will get both of them to experi-ence small signs of appreciation. This is also an area in which we can al-low ourselves to reach beyond solution-focused ideas and resort to sug-gestions that interrupt patterns or externalize the symptom (White & Epston, 1990). The goal is to perturbate so it fits the client as much as possible. Because every client is different, the decision about how to perturbate requires broad thinking. The ideas we come up with must al-ways consider the clients' way of cooperating. For example, if a couple is highly competitive, one may tag the end of the suggestion with a com-ment such as "I wonder which one of you will have the strength to risk showing appreciation first?"

When designing suggestions it is also important to keep in mind that *SFT goes slowly*. Clients who have been immersed in a problem for a long time may need time to ready themselves for change, even if it is positive.

Following are four questions solution-focused brief therapists may find useful when formulating suggestions:

1. How did the client describe the situation? (content)
2. What did the clients want? Is he or she willing to change?
3. How do the clients act about what they are saying?(process)
4. How can the different information or perspective provided in the summation message be translated into a suggestion?

Case Example (Continued)

The B family members' description of the problem:

Mom—Tina has behavior problems.
Dad—Tina has behavior problems.
Mike—I don't want to be involved.
Tina—Things are not good at home and at school.

What do the clients want?

Mom—Tina should listen to adults more.
Dad—Tina should be happier.
Mike—Everyone should be happier.
Tina—Mom and Dad should be happier with me.

How are the clients responding to the situation? Are they willing to do anything different?

Mom—Keeps looking for something to change Tina.
Dad—Keeps looking for something to change Tina.
Mike—Ignores the situation
Tina—Does nothing.

It is uncertain as yet whether the parents and Tina will do something different. Their reaction to the suggestion will provide more information about that.

How can the difference presented in the summation message be translated into a suggestion? The message was different in that it affirmed everyone. It highlighted their common desire for happiness in the family. It may be best to try to continue the process of focusing on exceptions and positives.

Suggestion:

"Unfortunately, we don't have any magic answers for you today. We are going to have to get to know you all a little better. We do have some suggestions that may help toward that end. We heard your concerns, and they are important, but we would also like to know a little more about what is working in your family, now that we know what some of the problems are. We want to be sure not to change any of that good stuff."

Separate suggestion to the parents because they are at odds:

"Mrs. B, if you get a chance, we would suggest you notice what Tina is doing at home and at school that you want her to continue to keep doing. Keep track of it so you can share it with us next week. [This is what Mrs. B said she wanted.]

"Mr. B, if you get a chance, we suggest you notice what is going on when Tina appears to be happier during the week. We'd appreciate hearing about that. [This is what Mr. B said he wanted.] You may want to compare your results with Mrs. B every evening and notice what you agree about.

"Tina, we'd like to suggest you try to notice what will be happening at school with the kids and teachers that you like and want to continue to have happen. If you want, you can do that about home, too. [Tina had said she wanted change at school.]

"Mike, if you feel like it, you could notice and let us know what will be happening in your family this week that you want to continue to have happen." [Mike seemed cautious about participating but is still given the choice to do so.]

In keeping with the assumption that *nothing is all negative,* and *clients have the resources to help themselves,* the family members were given suggestions to focus on their idea of solution rather than on the problem. The responses will be valuable, regardless of what they are, because they will provide further information about the family's style of cooperating.

Case Example: James

This is another example illustrating the use of these questions.

James said he decided to talk to someone because he felt desperate and was not able to help himself. Six months ago, at age 53, during a downsizing at his job, his position was eliminated His intensive efforts to find another job failed. James was increasingly plagued by the injustice of it all and had now stopped answering ads or sending out resumes. James's appearance reflected neglect, and he reported increasing desire to isolate himself socially. At the same time, he expressed anger and disgust with himself for his lack of energy and said that all he wanted was to be his old self again. He described his old self as a self-starter and positive thinker.

The first part of the summation message should reflect that the therapist heard and understood the events that brought James into therapy, and that he or she empathizes. The second part, the therapist's response, should reinforce James's strengths: his recognition that he needs help, his decision to follow through on it, his sense of justice, and his history of thinking positively and being proactive. It should also offer new information or a new perspective. One idea that comes to mind here is to use James's sense of justice as a resource for another perspective.

Option A:

"While your anger about the injustice that led to your work situation makes a lot of sense, we notice that your anger at yourself for not having found work yet is very unjust. It is hard to have a positive attitude and self-start when one feels one is being treated unfairly. Unfortunately you cannot do anything to change your company, but we wonder whether you are interested in considering how you could treat yourself more fairly?"

Using the aforementioned four questions, here are two options for suggestions. There are certainly many other possibilities.

1. The client describes himself as stuck because he has no energy and is angry at others and himself. He proclaims that he wants help to change.
2. He wants to be like his old self again.
3. The client's response to the situation is anger at others and at himself. The angrier he gets the less control he feels.
4. The different perspective offered was that the client is being unfair to himself. His sense of justice is strong. Asking him to apply his sense of justice to himself may be a successful perturbation.

Option A:

"We have a suggestion, James, that some people have found helpful in situations like yours. It requires you to set aside half an hour twice a day, at the same time. During the first 15 minutes you would write about your anger about the situation and at yourself. The next 15 minutes you would think about and list ideas for treating yourself more fairly. At the end you tear up and throw away the first notes and keep the second notes."

Option B (This option uses James's anger):

"We are not surprised that you feel stuck because your anger at the situation, and at yourself, is sapping all your energy for self-starting. It seems to us that you may have to try to do something different to get your old, energetic, self back."

"We have a suggestion that might help you get unstuck and slowly accomplish that. Think of whether you might want to give this a try! It's going to take some time to get back to your old self, and to stop being angry. It's a little like changing a habit. So, we suggest that when you notice that you are angry that you figure out approximately how much time you need to get through that particular part of it. Say, you are really angry at yourself for not having sent in any resumes. Decide how many minutes you need to really get the anger out. When the time is up, spend half that time doing something else, preferably something your old self would have done. It can be anything except being angry."

Both these suggestions are behaviorally oriented as a way of cooperating with James's request for something he can do to help himself but address his emotions as well. It also seems to make sense to suggest a ritual because it provides structure and control.

Frequently Used Solution-Focused Suggestions

Most of the suggestions listed here belong to the systemic/strategic/structural tradition and are used so widely now that it is difficult to pinpoint their original source. They are suggestions originated by, or adapted from, those used at the Brief Therapy Clinic at the Mental Research Institute and those used by Jay Haley, Salvador Minuchin, the Milan Team, and the Ackerman Institute. However, the Formula-First Session Task and the Prediction Task originated at the Brief Family Therapy Center. It is important to remember that these suggestions, much like tailored ones, must fit the particular context of the situation to make a difference.

1. *Formula-First Session Task.* This suggestion can be given at the end of most first sessions except those that involve severe grief, loss, or a problem description that has no exceptions.

"Between now and next time we meet, we would like you to observe, so that you can describe to us next time, what happens in your family that you want to continue to have happen" (Adams, Piercy, & Jirhc, 1991; de Shazer, 1985, p. 137).

In the aforementioned case of James, this suggestion does not fit because James's view of his situation is so negative. The suggestion may actually exacerbate James's anger at himself.

2. *Do more of what works.* This suggestion is guided by the idea of

not fixing something that is working already. It works well when presession change has been reported or already existing positives are evident.

3. *Do something different.* This suggestion is for clients who are eager to be told what to do and what they are doing is not working.

4. *Don't change.* This suggestion is usually effective when a situation is critical and clients want an immediate solution. It should not be used when clients are in danger of harming themselves or others.

> "We understand how serious this situation is, and how badly you want it resolved as soon as possible, but we feel we may not be able to be helpful without getting to understand things a little better. So, we suggest that you do not change anything until we meet again. When things are this precarious they could get worse and we don't want that to happen."

5. *Go slow.* This step is suggested when clients feel pressure to change, or when they are progressing well. It is helpful to tell people that good change takes time to take hold, so they should move ahead slowly. It avoids disappointment if progress is not steady.

6. *Do the opposite.* This is a good suggestion to give to one partner of a couple who is being seen alone, or to parents who are seen without their child, when repeated attempts to change another person has not worked.

7. *Prediction Task.* This suggestion is made when clients can report some exceptions to their problem but cannot explain why they happen. When this suggestion is given to a couple, or a family, the decision about whether to share the results before the next meeting depends on the particular case. With parents, if the goal is to get them to be more of a united front, it is appropriate to suggest they share results and discuss them every night with each other but not with the child. The child should do the prediction on his or her own and not share until the session. In the case of a couple where both partners believe the other does not care, it is best not to ask them to share until the session. There can be disappointment if nothing is shared one day, but chances are that there will be some pleasant surprises by the next session.

> "Before you go to bed tonight predict whether [the symptom, or the situation] will be the same or better tomorrow. [One can also ask clients to develop a numerical scale on which they can predict the degree of the problem for the next day.] Tomorrow night rate the day and compare it to your prediction. Think about

what may have accounted for the right prediction or the wrong prediction. Repeat this every night until we meet again and keep a record of the daily results" (de Shazer, 1988).

8. *Write and burn.* This is a good suggestion for people who are stuck in an emotional state that keeps them from functioning the way they want to. Some people do not like to write. One can suggest that they talk into a tape and erase the tape.

"Set aside 20 minutes twice a day [the time and frequency can be adjusted to the particular case] to write about your pain [anger, frustration, etc.]. Don't try to write carefully, just put the pen to the paper and let it flow. If you find yourself repeating phrases, or words, that's fine. Just get your feelings out. If you have to cry and scream along with it, that's OK, too. When the time is up, don't read what you wrote, burn it and watch it go up in smoke." [This can be suggested only by discussing with the clients whether they have a safe way of burning paper. If there is no guarantee of safety suggest they tear the paper up into tiny bits and watch themselves dropping it slowly into the trash can.]

CONCLUSION

It is evident that the formulation of the summation message and the suggestion is not easy. It is a true synthesis of what our clients are able to offer us and what we can offer them in terms of our professional knowledge and humanity.

In summary, it might be a useful exercise to rethink what kind of summation message and suggestion would have reflected the situation presented by Marie, in Chapter 3.

Marie was the single mother who felt misunderstood by everyone and was afraid she was crazy. She was referred because her physician could not find any cause for her physical symptoms.

Summation message:

1. A statement about what the therapist heard the client say:

"What we heard today is that you came because your doctor suggested it when you went to see him about pains in your whole body and really bad headaches. You said it concerned you that he sent you to talk to someone. Your fear is that he thinks there is something wrong with you mentally.

"We heard that you are separated from your husband and you and your two children are living with your mother. This is hard, because it's her house and she wants you to do things her way. Your ex-boyfriend and husband are also in and out of your life trying to tell you what you should and shouldn't do, which is really hard on you.

"We also heard that you have some clear plans about your future, like getting an education, and making sure your kids are well educated, but everyone is holding you back instead of helping you."

2. A response from the therapist that includes empathy, positives, and different information or perspective:

"Our response is that you are under a great deal of stress. No wonder you have headaches and all sorts of aches and pains when you keep all you have told us bottled up. We're surprised that you are doing as well as you are, given your life right now. It must be hard not having a place of your own and having people put you down for having different ideas than they do. And in spite of that you get along well with your children and continue to teach them and go to the library to educate yourself, and all that with so little sleep and so little support.

"You have some good ideas for the future, like a place of your own and applying for school, and you say that before anything you just need a little time to relax and have some fun, like going bowling. It is good that you realize that it is going to take some time to make those plans happen and you need to feel healthy and relaxed in order to do that."

The suggestion:

1. Marie described the situation as being anxious about her symptoms and feeling stressed because she has no support for achieving her goals. She implied she wants to change but not necessarily as a result of coming to therapy.

2. Marie wants to know whether there is something seriously wrong with her. She also wants to find a way to live her own life without interference.

3. Marie's response to her situation is to somatosize her stress and to keep pursuing her goals the best she can.

4. The different information she was given in the summation message is that she is not crazy and that she is doing well under the circumstances. This information should provide some relief in itself. The suggestion should offer more relief (e.g., the opportunity to vent her anger and frustration in a safe way).

Suggestion:

"We wish we had some magic answers for you today, but of course we don't. We'll have to put our heads together some more to see how you can begin to build that future. Meanwhile, we really don't think you need to worry any more about being crazy.

"We have a suggestion that you may want to think about, or not [echoing her way of speaking]. Because you can't tell the people who are upsetting you what you think, and it's upsetting you a lot, you might want to get it out another way. Some people find it really helpful to sit down for half an hour a day, at the same time, and just write out all their upset feelings. When they are done, they don't read it over. They just tear it up in little pieces and get rid of it. Even if you write the same stuff over and over it can be helpful. When you've done that write down three reasons why you are a good person and a good mother."

Notice how all the pieces of the solution-focused process fit together. The emotional climate facilitates the interview that generates information for the summary. The summary repeats that information, adds to it, and makes it experiential by means of a task.

Part II

Applications

8

Couple Therapy

Couple relationships are an excellent example of what structure coupling is all about. The biological, emotional, and economic interdependence of men and women has preserved our human race for thousands of years.

Working with couples—unmarried, married, heterosexual or same sex—can be like walking a tightrope. Couple relationships are complex; they are not just about chemistry and companionship. Couple relationships go through phases that usually start with romantic blindness and move through more and less difficult times of adjustment to realistic differences in personality, to changes in ways of living, and to shifts in mutual needs. Couple relationships have uncanny ways of becoming what one least expected or wanted them to be, at times even a replication of a relationship with a parent or a sibling. It is said that partners tend to complement each other to compensate for each other's weaknesses, but that complementary balance can lead to a power struggle as easily as it can enrich a relationship. Nevertheless, most people prefer to live in couplehood rather than to be single, regardless of the circumstances.

The importance of relational ties is a powerful resource for therapy. A question such as "What do you need from each other to feel just a little bit less (hurt, afraid, angry)?" can turn " 'hard' feelings into 'soft' emotions" (Donovan, 1999, p. 5; Gilligan, 1997; Johnson & Greenberg, 1994). "Soft emotions" is what couple relationships are all about, regardless of how tough or cold a client may appear.

Jane and Steve describe their relationship from different points of view:

127

JANE: Steve seems to be spending less and less time with me. I don't know what happened to our friendship. He used to discuss everything with me and ask my opinion.

STEVE: I don't think that's my fault. Since you started to run marathons your running always comes first. You don't have time for me anymore.

JANE: That's not true. I try to get you to talk but you just sit there and stare at the tube. (*to therapist*) What would you do if your husband started to ignore you?

STEVE: (*to therapist*) I don't ignore her. There's just no point in discussing anything with her because she has a chip on her shoulder and I can't say anything right. (*to therapist*) Am I supposed to just take it all?

The therapist cannot answer either question directed to her without taking sides. Moreover, responding to the content of these complaints is likely to lead to an adversarial exchange. However, the therapist can look for a common thread in what both partners are complaining about and use it as a resource to connect them:

THERAPIST: *You both* sound dissatisfied with the lack of attention from each other. (*Both partners nod and elaborate on that some more.*) *You both* seem to want the same thing. Was there a time when *you both* felt more satisfied with the attention you were getting from each other?

These questions draw Jane's and Steve's attention to the fact that they are still connected when they probably felt very disengaged. A *small change can lead to bigger changes.* If Jane and Steve had redefined their problem as "not enough time together" and worked out a solution that satisfied them both, some solution-focused therapists would recommend terminating treatment. My experience has been that these "miracle cures" do happen but are rare. They can bring clients back several months later with the same or a similar problem representing the same process. (In the language of systems theory, a "first-order" change occurred rather than a "second-order" change (Hoffman, 1981, pp. 47–49; Watzlawick et al., 1974, p. 10). This situation can be avoided by making the effort to anchor the changes more solidly. In this case, it would be to clarify with the couple what it is about spending more time together that will represent improvement for them. Chances are their answers will be in the emotional realm, about feeling more connected, more cared for, or more acknowledged. This clarification enhances their understanding about their relationship and can serve a valuable preventive function.

Basically, solution-focused work with couples is the same as with individuals (Friedman & Lipchik, 1999; Hoyt & Berg, 1998). However, what makes practice more difficult is that the solution has to satisfy the relationship, and the relationship consists of individuals with differing points of view. To overcome that hurdle both partners must trust the therapist not to take sides against him or her. Even for the most experienced therapist it can be a challenge to convey acceptance and understanding to two people who both believe they are right.

The following steps were developed to show ways to manage these complexities with a greater degree of confidence. The first step is to determine whether a couple is appropriate for solution-focused couple therapy.

THE ASSESSMENT

A Conjoint Session

The first session should be a conjoint session because it offers the therapist a sampling of how the partners interact with each other. It is also a way of gauging their desire and capability to work on the relationship. Solutions do not happen without people wanting to make them happen. Couple work, in particular, is unlikely to be productive when both partners do not have similar goals and are not invested in contributing to the solution. Thus a husband who wants to save the marriage at all costs and a wife who is not certain about remaining in the marriage would not be ready for solution-focused couple work. (It is rare, indeed, that an individual case is deemed inappropriate for SFT. One major exception may be clients who clearly do not want to be in therapy and have come only to please someone else.) In such a situation, it is better to discuss these differences with the partners in a separate session and to clarify their needs further. Sometimes an undecided partner needs a few individual sessions to come to a decision. During that time the committed partner may be seen separately as well, for support. If it appears as though an undecided partner needs a long time to make a decision, it is best to refer both partners elsewhere for individual work and invite them to come back for couple work if they both decide they want to work toward a better marriage.

In the first session of couple therapy, clients should be told that the contract for therapy is with their relationship, not with them individually, and that the goal will be to build a bridge between their differences that will lead to a solution for both of them. This makes it clear that the therapist will not take sides. Dual-track thinking that monitors our own reactions is helpful toward that end because it is often difficult to remain impartial. The acceptance and understanding of both sides can also be reflected in the summation message at the end of the session.

An Individual Session with Each Partner

The conjoint session is followed by a private one-on-one conversation with each partner. These conversations give the therapist the opportunity to develop the therapist–client relationship in more depth. At the beginning of this session the therapist tells the client that their private talk is an opportunity to discuss matters that he or she may not want to say in front of the partner. Confidentiality should be assured unless it concerns life-threatening information. If the client shares something that has important implications for the relationship the therapist must ask permission to share it.

The confession about an affair that ended in the past should be considered confidential information. Although it is significant in terms of the relationship, it is best not to base assumptions about the present state of the marriage on it. After all, *change is constant and inevitable*. It is more useful to stay focused on the present and what the client wants for the future.

Information about an ongoing affair is another matter. I do not work with a couple when one partner is involved in an affair. In general, people are not able to generate enough motivation to revive a less than satisfying relationship while participating in a more gratifying one. More important is the fact that such a secret represents a collusion with one partner that I consider unethical. A suggestion for handling such a situation is to tell the client having the affair either to share the secret or to discontinue any contact (including phone or e-mail) with the lover for the duration of treatment. I have actually been surprised about how many people choose to do this and stick with it. Of course, that says a lot about their motivation to improve their marriage! On the other hand, some people agree to put the affair on hold but do not follow through with it, and then there are the people who successfully deceive us. Generally, if a decision is made to work with the couple and the adultery continues there will be telltale signs such as no progress or fluctuations between progress and relapse. Therapists' intuition can also be a valuable tool.

I recall a situation in which the husband had agreed to end an affair. He appeared to be working hard to rekindle his relationship with his wife and she agreed that he was. However, she reported that she was not able to feel any changes in their emotional connection. I asked for separate session based on this information and the husband confessed he was continuing to meet with his lover. He said he was working on the marital relationship for the purpose of improving it so he and his wife would have less conflict around the children after he got a divorce.

In a situation such as this, it is advisable to tell the adulterous party that you will not continue working with him and his wife unless the truth is revealed. This proviso usually produces a crisis and places that partner in the position of finally having to choose between the marriage and the affair. The best way to terminate a case such as this is to meet with both partners and tell them that you have come to the realization that individual therapy would be more beneficial for them at this time. Such an announcement will obviously be met with questions by the partner who is oblivious to the continuing affair. In this situation only, I suggest assuming an expert position and sticking to a general statement without giving specific reasons. I also recommend offering referrals for individual treatment rather than continuing to see either partner.

In general, clients tend to reveal more in the one-on-one session than they do in the conjoint one, even those who start out by saying that there is nothing they would not say in front of their partner. Recently, I saw a couple who had some severe problems with extended family because of the wife's inability to get along with the husband's mother. In the conjoint session he never disputed his wife's story about his mother's unjust treatment of her. In the private session he spoke at length about his wife's problems with social relationships in general, not only with his family.

The use of circular questions that ask one partner what he or she thinks the other partner thinks, or why he or she thinks the partner acts a certain way, is a valuable resource in the private session. It can be considered a form of doing couple work with an individual because it requires consideration of the other person's perspective. For example, "Does your wife also believe she does not get along well with others?" "Have you talked with her about what you just shared with me?" If so, "What was her response?" If not, "How do you think she would respond if you did?" If he felt he would upset her too much, "How do you usually communicate things you want to tell her that may upset her?" Some clients have a sophisticated understanding of how they and their partner affect each other. Others are totally oblivious to interpersonal dynamics. The use of circular questions and other inquiries that address the clients' beliefs about the reasons and meaning of their partners behavior and their own responses to it are perturbations that may lead to change.

How clients respond to conversations that reveal recursive interactions with their partners also provides valuable information about how they cooperate. However, we must be careful not to make assumptions about how their manner of cooperating might affect the outcome of their therapy. After all, it is the couple that must decide whether a relationship is good enough for both of them! A small change that may seem inadequate to us may make a lot of difference to them.

The Decision

The decision about whether couple treatment is appropriate derives from the information obtained from the conjoint and two individual sessions. I use the following criteria as guidelines. It is too extreme to say that I follow them to the letter. There are times when we experience something about a relationship that tells us to try working with it in spite of some questions. We should not shut out that intuitive voice.

1. Both partners are clear that they want to stay in the relationship rather than leave it.
2. Both partners understand that they each has some responsibility for the quality of the relationship.
3. Both partners are able to demonstrate some empathy for their partner's position.
4. Both partners describe some positives in the relationship (friendship, mutual interests, ability to function well as parents or homemakers).
5. Neither partner is interested in another person, or engaged in an active affair with another person.

If it is clear that it is appropriate for the couple to work together, the next meeting scheduled will be a joint session.

Sometimes a couple meets all the criteria for couple work but is so hurt or angry that they cannot stop venting in each other's presence. In such cases I schedule one or two sessions separately to see whether I can help them drain off their feelings enough to work together productively. It also allows for an opportunity to gradually interject questions about what is working in the relationship.

THE THERAPY

Couples are usually upset when they first come to therapy and want to share all their most negative feelings. It is often hard not to be drawn into this negativity and to make assumptions about outcome. We must stay alert to the personal track of our dual-track thinking. Judgmental comments such as "Oh, this marriage is over!" can only lead to impasse and must be counteracted with *nothing is all negative* and *a small change can lead to bigger changes*. Similarly, we must counter any blame we notice ourselves ascribing to either partner with a reminder that their behaviors are recursive. "What is John doing that makes Mary decide to cut him down so?" "What makes John decide not to stop Mary from cutting him down?" Couples can also trigger personal associations in us about our parents' relationship, or our own. If we do not stay tuned in to our own thoughts and feelings we may develop a hidden agenda for clients without being aware of it.

Typically, partners try to convince therapists that their version of the situation is correct. It is important not to become part of that process. A good response is, "I expect you to have two very different stories and I need to hear them both so that I can help you build a bridge between them." This gives the message that they are not expected to change for each other. People tend to defend themselves again changing, particularly to suit someone else's expectations. It is, therefore, more palatable to use language that suggests stretching, growing or adapting, rather than changing.

Alternating Conversation with Each Partner

Another way therapists can maintain balance is to alternate talking with both partners. Frequently switching attention from one to the other prevents the partners from feeling slighted, and the therapist from feeling more connected with one person than with the other. On the other hand, we have to cooperate with the individual partners' styles. It is not unusual to find a verbally expressive woman coupled with a much less expressive man. Donovan (1999, p. 14) quotes Gottman and Levenson (1986) as saying that women are more able to regulate their affect in interperson conflict and therefore more often seem to take the complaining position, whereas their male partners withdraw to contain affect. All of us have also met couples whose dynamics are reversed. We have to remember not to try to level the field. It is sufficient to gently interrupt the expressive partner to ask the less expressive one, "Do you agree with this?" or "What do you think?" We then accept what is offered in order not to imply one style is preferable to another. The difference in expressive style may well be a problem in the relationship, and any sign of judgment about it could make one of the partners feel demeaned.

I had the opportunity to talk with a former client whom I treated with her husband in a domestic violence situation several years earlier. She reported that there had been no further episodes and that their marriage was much improved. When I asked what she thought was most helpful about our work together she replied, without hesitation, "The fact that you never took sides!" She could offer no further explanation about why that was helpful. Sprenkle, Blow, and Dickey (1999, p. 348) quote Pinsof's (1995) theory that the entire client system will have an alliance with the therapist that may be more than the individual and subsystem alliances combined. My own theory is that when two people in conflict become aware that their therapist, whom they trust, accepts their partner's views, it challenges them to rethink their own attitude.

How to Confront Gently

There are times when professional ethics demand that we confront a client's behavior. In SFT this has to be done in a manner that preserves the emotional climate.

Bill was sent to therapy by the district attorney's office as part of a diversion agreement instead of being charged. Neighbors had called the police when they heard him shouting threats at Ann during a fight. Ann had requested that they have couple work together, and this was agreeable as there had never been any physical violence.

During one session Bill was venting about a poor decision Ann had made recently. He used derogatory words such as "stupid" and "brainless." Aside from taxing a therapist's ability to stay impartial, it seems unethical to allow one client to verbally abuse another in a session. Ann admitted that she had acted impulsively and expressed regrets. This did not calm Bill down.

THERAPIST: You really can't understand how Ann could have made that decision. It makes you very angry. I can understand that. But, of course, it happens! We all do things at times that we wish we hadn't. (*Bill continues to vent anger.*) (*calmly*) Bill, have you ever made a poor decision?

BILL: Yeah . . . but not without thinking.

THERAPIST: But even one's thinking isn't always perfect. What kind of a reaction do you want from Ann when you make a mistake?

BILL: The same I'm giving her. She can yell at me! I'm already yelling at myself more than anyone else could yell.

THERAPIST: Ann, what do you think?

ANN: (*crying*) I'm hard on myself, too. I feel terrible, but I don't think you should kick someone when they are down.

BILL: (*blushing*) Well . . . you know how much this is costing us and how hard it is to earn money . . .

ANN: I know . . .

BILL: OK . . . OK . . . I shouldn't. . . . I'm sorry.

THERAPIST: In the future, when either one of you makes a mistake, what is the most helpful thing you can do for each other?

ANN: Not call each other names!

BILL: I guess to realize we're kicking ourselves already. No need to pour salt on the wound.

Instead of coaching Ann to stand up to Bill, the therapist chose to confront him in a gentle manner as a way of modeling behavior for Ann. Bill had a trusting relationship with the therapist who believed that Bill was likely to defend himself against any confrontations by Ann. Notice that the therapist first taps into Bill's own feelings to evoke some empathy. Thinking of Ann's feelings arouses some shame or guilt in Bill. To prevent these denigrating feelings from disturbing the emotional climate, the therapist shifts the focus from Bill to the couple's future, thereby emphasizing mutual responsibility in relationships.

Handling Conflict in Sessions

Couples describe their problems in words as well as in actions; therefore, they are likely to argue contentiously in sessions. This can be a particular dilemma for the solution-focused therapist, whose intent is to build on the positives in the relationship. On the other hand, couples' conflictual behaviors provide a valuable description of the problem.

How to handle arguing in sessions depends to some degree on when in occurs during the treatment process. In the first or second session, it is best to let it to go on long enough to get a sense of the pattern before interrupting it as gently as possible. Questions that come to mind include:

"How do you usually end fights like this at home?"
"Is this an example of what happens at home?"
"I'm wondering whether you want to use your time in the session like this?"

If the couple is having a conflict about something that happened in the past: "I know you both feel strongly about your opinion but we really can not change what happened in the past."

These responses usually stop the fighting but must be followed by a constructive focus to keep it from resuming. Given the intense negative emotions aroused by fights it is best not to ask about positives too quickly. This seems to have a rebound effect that leads to more negatives. It is more useful to ask what the fights mean to the couple. This will uncover new information that provides opportunities for solutions.

For example, in their first session, Tara and Sid, who both want to stop the incessant fighting in their relationship, interrupted each other constantly in spite of the therapist's effort to intervene. Consequently, their anger at each other continued to escalate. When the therapist asked them what their partner's anger meant to them it stopped the fighting. Tara said Sid's anger meant she could never do anything right. Sid said Tara's anger meant she could not tolerate any criticism. They both denied these interpretations, which gave the therapist the opportunity to shift into a constructive conversation about what they were angry about and how they could deal with it differently in the future.

When fighting breaks out at a later stage of treatment, when the clients consider themselves to have made some progress already, it is useful to ask the clients how they explain their inability to settle this argument in view of the positive changes that have occurred. Another option is to ask them how they can stop this argument in view of what they learned from the changes they have already made. If neither of these ideas work, it is best to speak to them separately to find out whether something is going on that they do not want to talk about in front of each other.

The procedure for dealing with fighting in session by couples who have a history of violence is to separate them and talk with them separately. The potential victim, usually the woman, should be seen first to ensure that she has a safety plan. If necessary, she can be helped to leave the office and seek shelter. However, the therapist then remains joined with the potential perpetrator by working with him on how he can keep himself safe from further criminal behavior. This preserves the therapist–client relationship with both partners.

Constructing a Unified Solution

Partners often describe their goals as seemingly different even though they both want them same thing from the relationship.

Fran and Sam both clearly stated they want to stay married and to feel close to each other again. They agreed that their first effort should be to communicate better, which meant less bickering to both of them. However, within minutes the couple was arguing whether they should discuss their finances or Sam's jealousy.

To avoid getting caught in this either–or process the therapist must help the couple redefine their view of the problem in such a way that it can bridge their individual views. An example would be to continue the conversation but replace the words "finances" and "jealousy" with "differences." Thus the conversation would become one of "bickering about differences" which they both agree on.

Another option is to switch to questions about when Fran and Sam "feel more connected." This is something both clients said they wanted and is certainly another perspective on their goal.

Still another option is to go a step further and introduce process in terms of a problem the clients have not stated themselves. "I'm wondering whether what you are both saying is that you feel controlled by each other?" If the couple agrees, the interview can continue with questions about what will be a sign to Fran that Sam is just a little less controlling financially and what will be a sign to Sam that Fran is just a bit less controlling with her jealousy? Are there times when they already feel less controlled by each other in those areas?

This example illustrates that, at times, therapists must contribute their own ideas, like their view of the process, to help clients focus their thinking. These contributions, when they fit for clients, are much appreciated and enhance the emotional climate, because they convey understanding. However, even if the idea is not accepted it can trigger clients' own thinking toward different and more helpful descriptions of their problem. For example, Fran and Sam might think that "controlling" each other is a less accurate description of how they feel than "being treated like a child." The clients' language is always best.

For clients to achieve what they want from therapy, they have to take responsibility for change and do something different. One telling sign that this is not happening is a report from one or both partners that things are deteriorating after having improved. This news is best explored in separate sessions with the partners. Sometimes the therapeutic process makes people realize that their expectations were wrong. Their partner may be fulfilling the expectations but their feelings have not changed. People can fall out of love when things have gone badly for a long time, and the old feelings can no longer be revived.

Communication

Most couples who come to therapy list "poor communication" as one of their major problems. This is usually their way of saying they feel misunderstood by their partner for what they say and do. A way of cooperating with this concept is to say "they have to learn each other's language." "Language" in this context means how people express themselves verbally and nonverbally. Clients are often surprised that love alone does not lead to understanding. The therapist builds a bridge of understanding by asking for clarification about each partner's words or actions. This puts their differences, which were formerly seen as lack of caring, in a more positive light and makes room for mutual adaptation.

Case Example: Miriam and Nate

Miriam left Nate a few months ago and recently returned to try to make the marriage work. The theme discussed here is their sexual relationship. Miriam felt pressured for sex by Nate, and Nate felt Miriam either rejected or avoided his sexual advances.

THERAPIST: Can you imagine any way Nate can initiate sex without you feeling pressured?

MIRIAM: Well, maybe if he used a more gentle approach . . . the whole thing . . . the timing . . . the "hey, how about it" . . . it's so . . .

THERAPIST: Are you saying you want him to be more romantic? (*Notices that Miriam and Nate exchange glances. Nate laughs in a sheepish manner.*)

MIRIAM: (*angrily to the therapist*) You see how he treats me. He laughs when I say what I need!

NATE: I wasn't laughing.

MIRIAM: Yes, you were. You do that a lot.

THERAPIST: What did you intend that laugh to mean, Nate?

NATE: I don't know. I get so frustrated because I just feel I can't win. I can't do it right for her, so I get frustrated.

THERAPIST: Are you saying you laugh when you feel frustrated?

NATE: Maybe! I never thought about it that way.

THERAPIST: Did you know that, Miriam?

MIRIAM: No. That doesn't make sense. When he laughs at me it just hurts me terribly.

THERAPIST: What are you hurting about?

MIRIAM: That he doesn't care about me, and what I want.

NATE: That's just how I feel. Last night I came in and she was on the phone, and I kissed her, and she shrugged me off. . . . (*Miriam starts to cry softly while Nate talks.*) Every time I try to show love there is rejection . . . so how can I continue to be romantic? Maybe I compensate by being angry, or critical. . . . I know I get that way . . . but what about my anger?

THERAPIST: (*to Miriam, who is still crying*) You seem very discouraged.

MIRIAM: I am. I'm trying to do my best to make our marriage work and it's never good enough.

THERAPIST: Let me understand this. Nate just said he tries to do things like kiss you when he comes home . . .

MIRIAM: (*interrupting*) When I'm on the phone? I'm not going to stop talking to have sex with him.

THERAPIST: (*to Miriam*) Is that what the kiss meant to you? That he wants sex?

MIRIAM: Yeah.

THERAPIST: (to Nate) Is she right?

NATE: No. This is a perfect example of what makes me feel rejected.

THERAPIST: (to Nate) What was the intention of that kiss?

NATE: I just came in the house and wanted to show her I was happy to see her. Every time I kiss her I'm not initiating sex.

MIRIAM: And I was arguing with my mother and didn't want to pay attention to him. He interprets everything I do as I don't love him.

NATE: (tearing) It's not that easy to trust you love me just because you came back. How do I know you really mean it unless you show it in your actions toward me? I'm always scared you'll leave again so I'm looking for reassurance. Don't you think it hurts me when you don't understand what I need? It really was good to see you cry now. It made me realize that maybe you do care. I don't want to hurt you . . . really!

THERAPIST: So are you saying, that everything you do is an effort to get reassurance that she loves you?

NATE: Yes.

THERAPIST: Is there some way she can reassure you of that even if she doesn't want to be touched or have sex at the same time you do?

NATE: She could say it! Well, sometimes she tells me she loves me . . . but not enough. I need to hear the words and then I don't have to try so hard in other ways.

MIRIAM: (to therapist) I didn't know that he was feeling this bad and that I don't have to take it so . . . so literally . . . whatever he does. I can remember that the next time, and reassure him instead of pulling away. But it would be easier for me if he told me what he's feeling, too. I'm not a mind reader.

Notice how the therapist literally acted as a translator for the couple, and in the process they learned to understand each other's intentions better.

Psychoeducation

A frequent argument among solution-focused brief therapists is how much coaching or teaching one should do to be truly "solution-focused." My answer is that if, as a result of our inquiries, we find that clients are obviously lacking some skills or information, we should seriously consider giving that information if we believe it will help the clients.

Sprenkle and his colleagues (1999) have remarked on the reluctance of postmodern therapists to offer information to clients.

> They might also be reluctant to see what they do as teaching or training. Still, helping clients, for example, to "re-author" their life stories, contains an instructional element. We believe that the imparting of information is probably a larger part of what most MFTs [marital and family therapists] do than is customarily recognized. (p. 344)

They also point out that an analysis of tapes of Minuchin and Whitaker showed that a high percentage of their responses could be categorized as providing information, interpretation, and guidance (Friedlander, Ellis, Raymond, Siegel, & Milford, 1987).

A useful concept to offer couples is developmental stages of relationships. Most couples expect their relationship to stay the same as it was when they first met, or even to get better. This is an unrealistic expectation. In the first stage of a relationship, the romantic stage, couples are "blinded by infatuation" and really do not know each other at all. They try to be what the other person wants them to be and minimize anything they do not like. Once some trust is established, they relax and behave more naturally. This is either accepted by the other or creates distrust and distance. Couples can be stuck at this point for years. The task now is to transition into the stage of emotional intimacy. This is a stage in which the real relationship begins and can grow forever. It entails being interested about differences rather than trying to eliminate them, and not trying to influence the other person to change. It means validating the other person by acting in a manner that conveys "I accept you and love you in spite of our differences," as opposed to "I love you only when you are who I want you to be." Differences are normal because everyone is unique, and in a healthy relationship they must be negotiated so that there is not a winner and a loser. Emotional intimacy means that partners are as interested in the other's happiness as their own and strives to achieve that.

This type of "education" is a form of reframing. Teaching people to communicate more clearly by offering specific skills is more direct teaching:

SUE: How many times can I ask you to call me and make sure I don't need something from the store before you come home from work?

FRED: When I get caught up with something at the end of the day all I think about is rushing home because you want me to help with the kids.

SUE: (*angrily*) What kind of help is that when I have to run out to the store to buy milk? Can't you think about me for a change?

FRED: (*increasingly angry*) I could say the same thing.

In a situation such as this it would be helpful to find out whether the couple is aware of different ways of communicating which are less likely to lead to anger, and whether they ever use them. If so, under what circumstances? What is different about those times? However, if they say this is their usual way of communication it is acceptable to suggest alternatives, such as "I" messages.

Sexual Intimacy

Sexual intimacy is an inherent part of any couple's relationship. Many couples feel free to address it on their own. Others do not talk about it until the therapist raises the subject. My own feeling is that clients want to talk about it and expect the therapist to ask about it. Generally, partners who are hurting in relation to each other report a decline in sexual frequency and satisfaction. Women, more than men, say they do not feel like having sexual contact when they feel hurt by their partner. Helping a couple restore sexual intimacy is a major link in bridging differences but one of the last ones to tackle unless both partners see it as a priority. Sexual intimacy requires a great deal of trust. When a relationship has been hurtful for some time it is best to rebuild or reinforce trust on other levels before risking a disappointing sexual experience.

Sometimes partners report that their sexual relationship is satisfying although nothing else in their relationship works. This information can be a valuable resource. It can be used to help the couple transpose some skills for satisfying each other sexually to other aspects of their relationship. One might say:

"Good sex requires subtle communication about giving pleasure and asking for what pleases. You two seem to be very skillful in that respect. What is it you do to show sensitivity to each other when you make love? What is different about how you feel about each other when you are making love than at other times?

[One should get as much detail as possible without making the clients uncomfortable.] What would be an example of using these skills in dealing with your (financial, parenting, bickering, etc.) problem?"

The Summation Message

Several points need to be emphasized in relation to summation messages for couples:

1. Be sure to tell each partner separately what you heard them say.
2. Respond to them separately, and be sure to include what you see their interactional process to be. "It is my impression that the two of you have different ways of reacting to feeling hurt. Mary lashes out and Jeff withdraws."
3. Tell them as many things as you can that you find they have in common. They do not have to be positive. They can include the intensity of their anger, their feeling of hopelessness. If nothing else point out that they both agreed to come to the session.
4. If they mentioned their feelings comment on that in "what I heard you say." If they did not, be sure to include something you sense about their feelings in "my response is."

CONCLUSION

Couple work is a careful balancing act to make sure we are conveying acceptance and understanding to both partners. To reinforce that our contract is with the relationship, not an individual partner, it is wise never to allow one partner to tell tales about the other over the phone between sessions. Be firm about discussing everything in front of the other partner in the conjoint sessions. Likewise, if one person asks for a separate session, be sure to inquire whether the partner knows about the request. If not, insist that the person tell his or her partner about the call and the reason for it. Always ask the other partner to come in for a separate session as well, to avoid any sense of partisanship.

Couples become families. The relationships between parents and children and siblings are different from those of two adults who have romantic ties. Therefore, family therapy is treated separately in the next chapter.

9

Family Therapy

Couples are unrelated adults who chose to be together and generally have legal means to end their relationship. Families have immutable ties that span generations. Parents are biologically motivated and socially mandated to care for their children until they are able to care for themselves. However, family relationships do not end when children become independent. Under the best of circumstances family members accommodate to the demands for different boundaries and changing connections. Under the worst circumstances, unresolved struggles cast inescapable shadows. Regardless of the quality of the family relationships, most cultures consider it an ethical obligation for adult children to care for their aged parents and/or siblings when they are no longer able to care for themselves. These ties that bind cast work with families into a different light than work with couples but are also a huge resource.

The therapeutic principles outlined in the previous chapter on couple therapy apply to family work as well. This chapter describes only the major differences.

ASSESSMENT

Assessment of families, unlike couples, is not to determine whether family therapy is appropriate. Because families cannot divorce each other and parents do not terminate their parental rights under any but dire circumstances, it is never a question of continuing or ending a relationship.

144

There will always be a relationship. The issue is the quality of the relationship and who is willing to participate in improving it. The purpose of the assessment is to establish whom to invite to sessions and in what groupings.

FAMILIES WITH CHILDREN OR ADOLESCENTS

The decision whether to involve children and adolescents in family therapy from the start is usually one based on theoretical orientation. Systemic therapists may prefer to see the entire family system *in vivo* in order to decide which patterns to interrupt or how to change the family's structure. They want as much information as possible about the system, from as many perspectives, including that of the 3-year-old who has not learned to edit stories (Minuchin & Fishman, 1981; Napier & Whitaker, 1978).

Therapists of a constructivist orientation are more likely to leave the choice of who wants to come to the session up to the family. This is in keeping with a nonexpert, accepting stance toward clients.

Naturally, the more family members with whom the therapist interacts, the more opportunities there are for solutions. On the other hand, change requires motivation, so that there is much to be said for having only the most motivated family members attend. Children can be disruptive in sessions, not only a source of valuable input. Parents may have pertinent information they cannot, or do not, want to reveal in front of young family members. Therapists may vary in their opinions about how much privileged information there should be in families.

My personal preference is to try to protect young people in their formative years from seeing themselves as defective, as they do when they have to see a "shrink," or from getting unnecessary labels. Because it is the natural order in the world for parents to help their children, and to teach them how to function in relation to others, it seems appropriate to begin by talking to them first about the situation. If they prove to be motivated to do something different themselves, goals can be met promptly and without ever having to involve the child. However, when parents see the problem as belonging to the child, as they often do, it is best to cooperate and evaluate the child as well before starting family sessions. Cooperating with parents is important because they have the power to discontinue therapy.

STRUCTURING THE CONVERSATION

A natural way to start the conversation, after some socializing, is to address family members in hierarchical order starting with the parents and ending with the youngest child. To avoid showing any gender bias I look at both parents at the same time and ask, "So who wants to tell me a little about your family and about yourselves?" This question will probably lead into their description of the complaints. One must always be sure to get both parents' stories regardless of who speaks first.

The next step is to look at both parents again and to ask what they hope will happen as a result of the sessions. This question leads to their ideas about goals. Here again, it is useful to check back and forth between the parents. I wait until the parents are finished to ask the children for their ideas about the problem and goals. More often than not parents and their children agree on the existence of conflict but not about the causes of it. Generally, preadolescents are more likely to concede that they need to change their behaviors. Adolescents, on the other hand, either feign diffidence or complain about the injustices they are experiencing in their life. These reflections of developmental issues should not tempt us to ignore them or forget that *every client is unique.* Young people can contribute a lot of valuable information to sessions if they feel safe and understood.

A cardinal rule when working with families is not to talk about differences too long without focusing the conversation on what the family members share, even if it is negative. Teenage children and their parents, in particular, perceive a deep abyss dividing them on all issues. They often describe their relationship as being like that of strangers, who have nothing in common, or enemies fighting a war. True, the job of allowing a child to become independent while still offering protection is a hard one. On the other hand, figuring out who you want to be other than what your parents want you to be and still wanting their approval and support is not easy either. The discovery that family members of all ages share anxiety, fear, and disappointments, as well as loyalty, love, and concern, can provide a good foundation for solutions. The change from an either–or view to one that is both–and triggers options.

CASE EXAMPLE: THE T FAMILY

The following case excerpt illustrates assessment and structure of a first family session.

Mr. and Mrs. T came with their two sons, Ron, 14, and Bob, 12. They were referred by the school counselor because of Ron's defiant behavior and some recent truancy. Mrs. T was adamant that the whole family should attend the session.

THERAPIST: (*addressing the parents after introductions and some socializing*) So, do you want to tell me a little bit more about what brought you here today? I understand the school suggested you come.

MRS. T: Well, Ron is giving us a lot of grief lately. I don't know what happened to him. He used to be such a good kid. No problems at school . . . B-plus student . . . nice friends . . . and now the grades are horrible . . . he's sassed some teachers and skipped classes. (*tearing*) I am really concerned.

THERAPIST: I can certainly understand that. . . . (*to Mr. T*) And what are your thoughts about all this?

MR. T: Well, I don't like it either. But I'm not as upset as Lily. I mean . . . it's unacceptable behavior on one hand, but I guess boys will get out of hand sometimes. I . . . I remember at that age I was. . . .

MRS. T: Oh, and what would your father have done if you had broken into people's mailboxes?

MR. T: Well, you know my dad. The belt came off right away, but these are different times.

MRS. T: (*to the therapist*) We found out from one of Ron's friend's parents that some of the boys have been into people's mailboxes and stealing things. (*She diverts from the school problem.*)

THERAPIST: What kind of things?

MRS. T: Magazines . . . stuff they shouldn't be looking at. . . . They got this idea . . . you know, we monitor what they're doing on the Internet . . . so they're sending for porno using the address of some of our neighbors who work all day, and then they take it out of the mailbox before the people get home. Sometimes they take other stuff they see there. . . .

THERAPIST: Like?

MR. T: I told him it's a federal offense. . . . Good thing they aren't stealing checks. . . . They've taken other catalogues and some ads for contests to win money.

THERAPIST: [Did not want to hear one side for too long and turned to the son for his version of the problem.] (*to Ron*) So, Ron. What's your side of this?

RON: (*Shrugs.*) Yeah. That's it . . . but we didn't do any harm. We don't take anything . . . or nothing valuable.

THERAPIST: Well, I'm also wondering what you think about what your parents are saying about all this, the mailboxes, and the changes at school . . . your grades? [Looked for the most open-ended way to assess what Ron considered the problem to be.]

RON: It's just not interesting anymore. It's boring.

THERAPIST: [Tried to understand and accept.] Hmm . . . yes . . . things do begin to feel a lot different at your age. Interests change. Do you have any concerns about what your parents are saying here today?

RON: Sure, but nothing's going to happen. I'm passing all my classes. . . . I want to go to college . . . and we've stopped that mail stuff.

THERAPIST: (*staying positive*) Well, I'm glad you are thinking of the future. Sometimes young people your age are too immature to consider the consequences of their actions for the future. (*to Mr. and Mrs. T*) Did you know Ron was thinking about his future?

MRS. T: It doesn't seem like it.

MR. T: I guess not.

THERAPIST: I bet it is a relief to hear him say he wants to go to college.

MR. T: He's so intelligent. We want him to have all the opportunities he can. We want him to feel good about himself.

MRS. T: We want to do things to help him but he has such an attitude. We get discouraged.

THERAPIST: Ron, did you know your parents felt this way?

RON: Ugh . . . no . . . they're always mad.

THERAPIST: What does that mean to you when they are mad?

Mr. and Mrs. T. learned that Ron felt that to him, their anger meant they have given up on him and he could not change that anymore. Ron discovered that his parents felt he had given up on himself and they were helpless to change that. The therapist then moved on to talk with Bob.

THERAPIST: So what do you think about all this, Bob?

BOB: I don't know. I think it's stupid. There's just too much yelling at the house.

THERAPIST: [Used a circular question to check out how the parents responded to Ron's behavior.] So what happens in your family when your parents get upset about your behavior, or Ron's?

BOB: Oh, they ground us or take away the phone. He gets grounded a lot . . . and Mom and Dad yell.

THERAPIST: (to Mr. and Mrs. T) Is grounding helpful?

MRS. T: No, not at all.

MR. T: I keep telling Lily it's too much. Grounding for a month at a time is too much. [The therapist did not respond to this disagreement between the parents at this time so as not to lose focus.]

MRS. T: Well, taking away the phone didn't work.

RON: If they'd just lay off I'd be all right.

THERAPIST: [Cooperated with the parents to establish the natural hierarchy but tried to stay connected with Ron, as well.] I know you believe that Ron, but they wouldn't be responsible parents if they didn't care about what's going on in your life. They're also legally responsible for you if you commit a criminal offense. But you seem to feel confident that things will be OK at school even though you're bored and that you won't go into mailboxes anymore. Any ideas how you can convince your parents of that?

RON: They'll just have to wait and see. I'll do better at school. . . . I am already.

MRS. T: If we could only trust that!

RON: You don't give me a chance. You treat me like a baby. You call the school, and my friends' houses.

MR. T: Lily gets real anxious . . . she's a worrier. She and her sisters never did anything wrong when they were kids at home.

THERAPIST: Do you trust Ron will stay out of trouble now?

MR. T: Well, not really. He's said he'll try before. Things have gone too far now. (Father sounds motivated.)

THERAPIST: So do you have any ideas about how Ron can prove he means what he says?

MR. T: Well, not really until we get a report card, or he isn't reported to be near any mailboxes. I think he should stop hanging out with the kids he did it with.

RON: (*angrily*) You can't blame them . . . it's not their fault.

THERAPIST: So, Ron, what's going to make you keep your word?

RON: They should leave me alone . . . not check on me. . . .

THERAPIST: At school? . . . in the neighborhood?

RON: She should stop asking me what happened at school . . . how much homework do I have? . . . did I do it? . . . where am I going?

THERAPIST: What do you think about that, Mom and Dad? [Addressed both parents, although Ron suggested that Mother had to stop pressuring him.]

MRS. T: Well, what if I did that and things got worse? And I think we should know where he is when he's out.

THERAPIST: (*agreeing with Mr. and Mrs. T*) Yes he should.

MR. T: I'm willing to let him show us that he can do it.

MRS. T: . . . and not tell us where he's going?

MR. T: No, I meant the schoolwork. We have to know where he is.

RON: None of the other guys have to check in. . . . I feel like a baby.

THERAPIST: (*cooperating with both Mr. and Mrs. T and Ron*) Ron, most parents who care expect to know where their kids are. So, Mom and Dad, Ron says he'll take responsibility for his behavior and work at school if no one monitors him. But it is always good to start with small steps. Ron, can you come up with a small step your parents can count on your doing at home and at school?

Ron showed motivation by saying he would show his parents his finished homework every night if they stopped asking him about it, and that he would check in after school to say whether or not he was coming home and where he would be. Ron and his parents were asked to come in separately. Ron was seen weekly for three sessions and then once 2 weeks later. His parents were seen twice, 2 weeks apart. Bob was not included. Ron was supported in making choices for himself that would benefit him in the long run, and in following through with his suggestions. Mr. and Mrs. B were helped to think of Ron's changes as small steps that needed to be reinforced rather than criticized. When both Ron and his parents reported progress at home and at school the family was seen together again, including Bob. Everyone could contribute ideas about what was different and how to continue making that happen.

PARENTS WHO DO NOT WANT TO BE INVOLVED

Some parents bring their child to therapy expecting him or her to be "fixed." They have no intention of participating in the process, which may be a sign that they feel defeated and have lost all confidence in their parenting. The best way to cooperate is to see the child alone and to engage the parents in therapy as consultants. In that capacity they feel safer and may gradually recognize the value of their participation. If they are reluctant even to do that, one should make an effort to get them to come in at least once "so I can get your side of the story."

The first thing to do in such a "consultation" is to listen for anything that can honestly be reinforced. One should never be insincere, like complimenting a parent for being consistent when he or she is only consistent occasionally. One can, however, say, "I can really tell how important it is to you to be a good parent! You are making an effort to be consistent about setting limits, and that is an important thing to keep doing." Such a statement is more likely to build confidence than a comment that the client knows not to be true. Confidence goes hand in hand with the courage to do something different. Joint sessions should not be suggested until the parents are assessed to have changed their attitude about a joint session.

When parents are clear that they do not want any involvement, the only option is to work alone with the child.

MEETING ALONE WITH THE CHILD

Meeting alone with children has the advantage of allowing the therapist to cooperate more closely with them than in the presence of parents. Parents expect the therapist to be their advocate. However, even without parents in the session it is still a difficult balancing act to accept the young person's point of view and to help him or her accept reality.

Young people usually want their parents to "get off their back" about something. Thus, complaints about parental requests or prohibitions must be countered in a kind but realistic manner, as demonstrated in the foregoing case. Suggesting to the young person that he or she do what the parents want is likely to undermine trust. To cooperate, the therapist can ask, "What is the least you are willing to do to get your parents off your back?" This offers an option that gives some control and is more likely to be considered supportive.

At other times children have parents who for reasons of their own are neglectful or uncaring. That makes it a painful but necessary task to help such youngsters grieve unrealistic expectations and mobilize their own resources to value themselves. The following case illustrates the latter situation.

CASE EXAMPLE: TROY

Eleven-year-old Troy was referred to therapy by a county program for delinquent youths in which he was participating after school. He and three other boys had been charged with trespassing and larceny for breaking into a house and stealing a TV and some money. The usual procedure for referrals from this program was that parents accompany the client for the first session and attend family sessions whenever the therapist recommends them. Troy's mother was curt and cold when the therapist called to schedule an appointment and refused to attend the intake session with the excuse that she had no one with whom to leave the younger children. She reluctantly agreed to a brief telephone interview during which she made it clear that she had washed her hands of Troy because he had just gotten worse over the years. She told the therapist she divorced her first husband when Troy was 2 years old. Her husband was an alcoholic who beat her, and he subsequently landed in jail for assaulting a policeman. She married her present husband when Troy was 4 and had three children with him. She was pregnant again and expecting another child in 2 months. She described Troy as "a handful" since he was born. She had taken him to therapy on and off since he was 4 to deal with temper tantrums, lying, and rebellious behavior.

Troy was a dark, handsome boy, who looked older than his age and was sprouting premature fuzz on his upper lip. He spoke up freely and had good eye contact. He readily admitted to the criminal behavior but rationalized it as the only way he could get any money because he was too young to work and his parents did not give him any allowance. He described his stepfather as a harsh, verbally abusive man and was very angry that his mother had never protected him from that abuse. "She thinks I'm a loser, just like my dad because he's in jail," he said.

Troy, unlike many boys his age, did not seem to mind coming to therapy. The therapist moved slowly at first to establish a relationship. She spent a number of weeks doing nothing more than making small talk, chatting about his passion, cartooning, and hearing his stories about his unhappy home life. Whenever the opportunity presented itself the therapist would compliment Troy for something. For example, when he reported one day that he had just cut one class that day instead of the usual three or four, she complimented him for having made that decision and wondered what other good things he had done for himself since they last met. When he reported walking out of the house once rather than engaging in a verbal battle with his stepfather, the therapists questioned him in detail how he had made such a good decision. At all times she listened with a "constructive ear" (Lipchik, 1988b) for anything that could be reinforced as good decisions and strengths.

Troy came faithfully and seemed disappointed when winter weather or holidays forced him to skip a session. When the therapist began to notice trust building she began to talk with him about what he wanted to get out of their sessions. Troy seemed taken aback by that question at first and said it just felt good to talk. The therapist explained the purpose of their meetings and asked him to come up with some ideas about what he wanted to work on.

TROY: I thought about it . . . what I want. I guess I want to learn to talk with my Mom the way I talk with you.

THERAPIST: Just Mom?

TROY: Well, I'm not sure about him [stepfather], but it would be nice if she could listen sometimes.

THERAPIST: Well, I think that is a really good goal, but you know, she may not have time to come in with you, and sometimes one person can't learn to have a good conversation with another person all by themselves.

TROY: So we can't try?

THERAPIST: Yes, we can try. I just can't promise you that if you make an effort to learn that she will respond the way you want her to.

TROY: That's OK.

THERAPIST: Well, can you remember any times when you had the kind of conversation with Mom that you are looking for? Even if it was just a little like that? [Troy could not come up with any exceptions related to his mother but was able to describe good conversations with his deceased maternal grandfather, a teacher, and an adolescent neighbor.] Why do you think you have better conversations with these people than with your mom?

TROY: I don't know.

THERAPIST: Is there anything different about you when you talk to them?

TROY: Yeah. It's like I have these two cartoon characters in my mind, a good guy and a bad guy, and they take over at different times. The bad guy is always the boss when I'm at home but never when I have a good conversation.

THERAPIST: Is that OK with you?

TROY: Yeah. They're bad guys so—the bad guy has to fight them.

THERAPIST: So in your cartoons, how do fights between bad guys end?

TROY: Someone has to end up good and the bad guys lose. But that won't happen at home. They won't become good guys and I won't either. My mom doesn't like me. She always says, "You're just like your dad, my real dad. You look like him, you act like him, and you'll end up like him.

The therapist began to have Troy draw cartoons about his good and bad guy in different interactions with other good and bad characters. The therapist also encouraged Troy to reach out to his teacher and the adolescent friend and have more good conversations with them. She helped Troy connect with his art teacher at school who, in turn, encouraged Troy to join the art club. As the "good guy" became more dominant in Troy's life and he began to feel better about himself, the therapist wondered whether the "good guy" would ever try to be dominant at home. Troy made some tentative efforts but he experienced them to make no difference in his mother's attitude toward him. This disappointment was discussed in therapy:

THERAPIST: I know you are disappointed. But you are really trying everything you can to have good conversations.

TROY: (*expletive*) . . . what's the sense of it all?

THERAPIST: Are you the only one your mother ignores?

TROY: No. She's always a crab, but it's worse with me. She just doesn't like me (*crying*).

THERAPIST: That's a very painful thought, but what does it say about you?

TROY: That I'm no good.

THERAPIST: Does it? How come there are so many other people who you have good talks with who think you're OK?

TROY: I don't know.

The therapist worked with Troy on the idea that he was a good person but that his mother may have problems of her own at this time that did not allow her to show her appreciation of him. Perhaps when he was older and she could see he is different than his father she would show how happy that made her.

Troy went through periods of anger and grief in adjusting to his mother's rejection. The therapist offered questions to ask himself when he felt angry or lonely: "What do I have to tell myself when my mom makes me feel like I'm no good?" "What do I have to do to take care of myself and not mess up because I feel I'm no good?"

Gradually Troy's behavior at school improved to the point that he was passing all his grades and did not act out as much. His mother continued to refuse involvement in treatment but the social worker on the case told the therapist that the mother said that Troy's behavior at home had improved.

The job of the therapist in a situation like this is to provide the support and tools for emotional independence. This does not mean seeing the child every week until he is an adult and making him dependent on the therapeutic relationship. It means helping him get his needs met outside therapy gradually, but being there for him when he needs support.

MEDIATING BETWEEN CHILDREN AND PARENTS

When a child confides that he or she is having a problem with a parent, the therapist must find a way to communicate that to the parent in an unthreatening manner and without compromising the child's confidentiality.

Children and adolescents frequently complain that a parent, often a single parent, is not available to them. The therapist can try to address this lack of availability in an individual session with parents but not without first giving the parent a chance to complain about the child and to express understanding about that. This puts the therapist in a position of being able to reflect that it must be hard to spend time with a child who makes one feel so defeated or angry. If this statement is accepted, it can lead into questions about exceptions. These questions may make the parent realize that things are better when he or she spends more time with the child. They can also provide the therapist an opening to talk about how children, in general, often improve with just a few minutes of undivided attention from parents. Sometimes parents are too angry to want to give more time, but once they have a relationship with the therapist there is a better chance that they may want to make some changes.

FAMILIES WITH AGING PARENTS AND/OR ADULT SIBLINGS

The percentage of older adults in our population is growing rapidly and will continue to do so in the future. Consequently, solution-focused therapists are consulted more frequently by caretakers of aging parents (Bonjean, 1989, 1996). Aging issues tend to be heavily laden with emotion because they entail a great deal of loss and anxiety for all the parties involved. The care of aging parents can raise unresolved parent–child and sibling issues, as well as creating new ones.

There are also times when adult siblings consult a family therapist to resolves problems between them. The basic theory and practice of SFT as described here apply to all these family problems, as well. Some particulars to consider are:

1. Remember to address both individual and shared feelings.
2. Remember that aging parents and their adult children are looking to maintain control over their daily lives as much as possible. A small change can make a big difference.
3. Think both–and instead of either–or.
4. For old parents and their children the focus on the future must be anchored in what can be maintained from the present, or re-

activated from the past. The assumption *you can't change the past, so concentrate on the future* has to be qualified when working with people who realistically face separation by death in the not too distant future. Thinking *nothing is all negative* or *people have inherent strengths to help themselves* is more helpful.

5. Make sure not to underestimate old people and treat them like children.

6. Monitor your own reactions carefully to avoid overidentification or pity. Help clients reach their goals, not yours. Keep reminding yourself that *every client is unique* and therefore every family situation is unique.

CONCLUSION

Working with families is often considered the most difficult type of therapy to do. It is difficult to try to join different people of different generations and to try to forge a connection between them at the same time. Regardless of how many family members attend a session, the whole family is always in the room in spirit, and the family therapist must be aware of them as individuals and their interactions with each other. Teamwork is a tremendous asset when working with families. When a team is not available, a break at the end of the session is imperative for the therapist to collect his or her thoughts and decide on a summation message and suggestion. Family therapy is also one of the most rewarding forms of therapy because, depending on the configuration of the family, there is always the potential that the solutions that are worked out in the present can generate to other families now and in the future.

10

Working with Involuntary Clients

Simon, a 34-year-old African American man, was ordered to go to therapy by the employee assistance program at his firm and placed on probation for 3 months. Noncompliance meant termination of the well-paid, managerial position he had worked himself up to in the past 12 years. The cause for his referral was an increasing number of complaints by his staff about his contemptuous, aggressive behavior toward them without reasonable cause. He was also reported to be drinking heavily.

My first impression of Simon was that he reeked of alcohol. He was in a belligerent mood and complained that he was being treated unfairly. Simon believed that his staff was trying to get rid of him because he did not tolerate laziness or poor work. Simon had become head of his department about a year ago and increased production by 45% during that time. Did he consider himself a hard taskmaster? He admitted that he might be, at times, but he simply could not understand why his staff could not accomplish simple tasks or make responsible use of their time. Simon believed that he treated people fairly and never held anyone to standards that he himself could not measure up to. He also vehemently denied excessive use of alcohol when I mentioned that it had been listed as a reason for referral.

Simon said he had agreed to come to therapy even though he disagreed with the complaints against him because he has a wife and two small children for whom he is responsible. When I wondered if there was anything that might be helpful for us to talk about he answered sarcastically, "How to get my wife to stop spending money like it was going out of style?" I answered that this would be appropriate if he felt it contributed to his overall stress. He could even bring his wife with him, if she wanted to come. Simon had a strong negative reaction to this suggestion.

We spent the rest of the hour discussing what would be a productive use of Simon's time as he had decided to comply by coming to therapy. It appeared as though the more I respected his opinion that he did not have a problem with anger, and the more I gave him freedom to choose a theme for therapy, the more he reflected on his behaviors at home and at work. By the end of the hour he decided that it might be of some use to him if he learnt to deal with frustration better.

Simon had obviously been drinking again when he came to the next session. He talked about an incident at work where one of is staff had repeated a mistake in a procedure he had reviewed with her just last week. He had been able to control his anger in her presence but he ruminated about it for the rest of the day. "Why did she do this to me?" he asked in an exasperated tone. How could he tell whether she was deliberately "doing it to him" or just hadn't learned the procedure well enough, I wondered. He answered that he had learned it in one day, and looked surprised when I asked whether he expects his staff to be as accomplished as he is. To Simon, success at work was about how hard one tried, not about being better than anyone else.

During the third session I noticed that Simon did not smell of alcohol quite as much. He seemed more relaxed, and started out by complaining about his wife. He was angry because she took the children out of the house almost every night after dinner. Frequently, she just went to a shopping mall and, in his opinion, spent money unnecessarily. He did not begrudge her their comfortable lifestyle but felt she was deliberately sabotaging his plans to secure their future. When he talked to her about this it led to conflict that was never resolved. Once again, he rejected my offer to deal with this problem in therapy.

Simon shared a painful memory from his childhood, which he said was triggered by my question about whether he expected others to achieve at his level. He related how rejected and inadequate he had felt in the second grade in primary school because he was never allowed to participate in the reading group circle. Instead, he was told to sit in a corner by himself with a different book than the group was reading. Now he realizes that he was separated from the group because he already knew how to read. He had taught himself at age 4. However, at that time it had felt like an unfair punishment, much like the mandated counseling felt like punishment for running his department so well. He also expressed anger at his staff for complaining about him instead of appreciating his goals, and for not cooperating with him.

I wondered whether Simon had any thoughts about his staff's motivation for their behavior. Did he have any suspicions that they were prejudiced? Simon related that he had felt the color of his skin made people reject him when he was a child, and that he was still sensitive to the injustices to which a black man was subjected in a white society. However, he did not think that race played a significant role in this particular situation.

For six more meetings we concentrated on constructive ways for Simon to handle anger when frustrated. He was gradually becoming more flexible in his expectations of others and had developed a more diplomatic managerial style. Sometimes he mentioned his frustrations at home but overall he seemed to manage better there as well. He still smelled of alcohol occasionally, but much less strongly than in earlier sessions. After 3 months of therapy he received an excellent evaluation from his department head. There was consensus among his staff and his supervisors that he had made significant changes in his behavior and that alcohol was not affecting his work performance anymore. I congratulated him on his good work and on having achieved his goal. To my surprise he answered, "Thanks, but now we have a bigger goal to work on!" He told me his wife had wanted to talk to me for some time now but he had not been ready. I explained that before conjoint sessions, I always have an individual session with the partner of a client I have seen for a while. Simon was agreeable to this.

Nancy, his wife, came in 2 days later and the first thing she said when she sat down was, "You know, Simon is an alcoholic." She said that Simon used to have a beer or two every night when they first met, but in the past few years his alcohol consumption had increased proportionately with his work responsibilities. It was so out of control since his last promotion a year and a half ago that she tried to leave the house when he came home from work to spare herself and the children his drunken hostility. He had cut back on his drinking during the past 3 months but she felt that it was still an issue that had to be dealt with. Nancy also felt there was work to be done on the relationship, particularly around finances and how to settle arguments, and that she needed to make some changes in that regard as well.

Nancy and Simon continued therapy for another 8 months. During that time Simon stopped drinking. He insisted on doing it "cold turkey." I was concerned about the possible complications without a medical intervention, but he was adamant. By this time I knew the value of cooperating with him. He did compromise and agree to hospitalization if his withdrawal became so difficult that it affected Nancy and the children adversely. In the end, Simon only suffered gradually diminishing headaches for about 6 weeks until he became comfortable with sobriety. He and Nancy agreed on some goals to work on to improve their relationship and felt satisfied with the results when they terminated.

Simon was a nonclient (hereafter referred to as "involuntary client") who chose to become a client. He not only met his own goals but those of his wife and his referral source. This is an ideal outcome but one not always to be expected. However, as this case demonstrates, with involuntary clients there is much to be said for cooperating, going slowly, and ensuring an emotional climate that promotes a trusting relationship. The use of solution-focused questions should be secondary until the client is motivated to discuss some goals for the meetings.

Some clinicians may disagree with my decision to have talked with Simon while he was intoxicated. In my experience, this is consistent with cooperating with the client and does not interfere with treatment in the long run. In Simon's case the drinking, particularly before coming to sessions, gradually diminished as he developed trust in our relationship. He addressed it when he was ready to do so, and he did it successfully. Had there been no change in the drinking pattern and no progress otherwise I would have referred him for alcohol counseling. However, clients are much more likely to stop denying after a trusting relationship has been established than when they first begin treatment.

WHAT DEFINES A CLIENT AS INVOLUNTARY?

The main reasons clients do not want to be in therapy is because they do not feel the need for it or because they are afraid of it. Typical examples are children whose parents bring them to therapy, people who are sent by their doctors, old parents whose grown children bring them, and clients who are mandated to come by their employers, like Simon, or by the judicial system because of antisocial behaviors.

Many involuntary clients think psychotherapy will make them feel worse because they will be told that they are crazy or bad. Others do not want to find out that therapy can help them because it would mean they were not good enough to help themselves. Clients sometimes fear they will never be able to stop coming if they agree to start. Many people have no better reason for not wanting to come than that someone else told them to do so. Most clients are clear about not wanting to be there from the start, but some pretend to comply until it becomes evident that they are not motivated to change.

On the surface it may seem that working successfully with people who do not want to be there is more difficult than working with voluntary clients. Certainly, the fact that self-referred clients already have some degree of motivation when they come is an advantage. However, as Turnell and Edwards (1999) point out, "the relationship is primary for successful outcome" (p. 33) with clients who do not want to be there. Because that relationship is guided by the therapist, the outcome is as much in the hands of the therapist as it is in the hands of the client.

THE THERAPIST–CLIENT RELATIONSHIP

Most involuntary clients are overtly or covertly antagonistic toward the person or system that referred them, and anyone associated with it. They experience them as intrusive and judgmental. Many clients undoubtedly want their situations to change for the better and may be willing to do something different to make that happen. However, they are usually given few choices about how and what to change and little encouragement for efforts that do not fit the expectations of those who are directing the changes. This combination of factors eventually leads to their being labeled "resistant" or "noncompliant," which reinforces the adversarial relationship between them and their helpers.

Agents of the law, social service workers, and mental health professionals are usually not malevolent and unfeeling. However, their relationship with clients depends on the demands and expectations of their jobs. Legal personnel must think of protecting the community above all; social service workers are generally overworked and do not have the luxury of tailoring interventions to individuals; mental health professionals generally consider clients' behaviors as pathological and are therefore intent on eliminating pathology in their clients.

The particular challenge of the solution-focused therapist–client relationship with involuntary clients is the need to connect with and meet the needs of both the clients and the referring person or system

(Rosenberg, 2000; Stanton, Duncan, & Todd, 1981; Tohn & Oshlg, 1996). It is difficult for clients to trust us when they perceive us to be agents of the courts or the social service system. On the other hand, referral sources are often not familiar with solution-focused philosophy and require extra time and patience to be familiarized with a process that is based on the belief that *a small change can lead to bigger changes* or *nothing is all negative*. It is difficult for us to balance a positive attitude toward clients and a cooperative connection with other professionals on the case without feeling triangulated at times.

Involuntary clients are also more likely to present long-standing problems that involve misfortune outside their control and/or antisocial behaviors. It can, therefore, feel like a stretch, at times, to believe *clients have the strengths and resources to help themselves* yet to maintain the hopeful and nonjudgmental stance clients need to recover their own strengths.

One of the most important aspects of the therapist–client relationship with involuntary clients is that they should experience the relationship as different from the one they usually have with professionals involved with their case. Establishing this difference takes time and does not happen until clients recognize that we genuinely care for them at the same time that we set professionally required limits.

Some examples of how to do that may involve mandatory reporting of child abuse, incest, or reoffenses by clients who are on probation or parole. Marilyn LaCourt (2001, personal communication) suggests that one way to protect the relationship is to ask the client to report the offense rather than the therapist doing it. This suggests to the authorities that the client is taking some responsibility for himself and places the therapist in a more neutral position.

In my work with spouse abuse, I try to act as both a therapist and an advocate for the victim and the perpetrator. Perpetrators must understand that I will not overlook a future offense, yet if tension arises between the perpetrator and his or her partner in a session, or is reported to be rising at home, I am as concerned about keeping the perpetrator safe from his or her own actions as I am about the victim's safety. The conversation with the potential victim is about an immediate safety plan; the conversation with the potential abuser is about how I can be helpful to him or her at this time so that he or she does not get involved with the authorities again.

However, when all is said and done, the message involuntary clients should get from their therapist is no different than the message any client should get. It is based on the assumption that *therapists can't change clients; clients can only change themselves*. It is clear that the therapist cannot change others, including the referral system, but it implies acceptance and support for the clients' effort to work on responsible solutions. Although this is no panacea, it often makes a considerable difference to clients who do not want to be in therapy.

COOPERATING WITH CLIENTS

Cooperating with an involuntary client whose goal is to avoid participating in therapy raises theoretical and ethical issues as well. Cooperating with involuntary clients is a therapeutic strategy developed to eliminate resistance and to convey acceptance to clients. When we cooperate with how the involuntary client cooperates (accepting that he or she does not want to be there) can we be thought of as siding with the client against the referring system, and if not, are we then using a strategy to get the client to comply with its demands?

Many therapists who choose to work with involuntary clients come to terms with these issues as a result of their altruism. For example, those who work in child protection reason that they want to keep children safe and living in their own homes, if possible. To that end they will cooperate with parents who may first deny purported physical or sexual abuse as long as the children are already safe. The Australian therapists Turnell and Edwards (1999) point out that cooperating does not mean accepting bad behaviors. "You cooperate with the person—not the abuse," and you "focus on what is expected—not what is wrong" (pp. 33–34). This focus builds trust and the sense of safety needed by clients to reconsider their own best interests, which ideally will also intersect with the goals of the referral source.

When working with spouse abuse cases my rationale for cooperating with batterers is, above all, to help women live safer lives with the men they choose as partners. Studies indicate that approximately 75% of women who have experienced battering return to their partners after a police intervention or a shelter stay (Feazell, Mayers, & Deschner, 1984; Purdy & Nickle, 1981). This seems a good reason to help couples improve their relationship under circumstances that have been assessed to be safe and appropriate (Lipchik, 1991; Lipchik & Kubicki, 1996; Lipchik et al., 1997).

When working with couples where one partner has abused the

other, therapists must be attuned to how both partners cooperate, just as in general couple work. (This is not to be misunderstood as accepting the point of view that abuse is justified. It means trying to understand the person's way of thinking and using his or her interactional style.) Turnell and Edwards's (1999) admonition that one can cooperate with the person without cooperating with the abuse is applicable here as well. In my experience, this approach to perpetrators has proven to be the fastest way to decrease denial and increase personal responsibility. Moreover, it contributes to the battered woman's safety. The batterer has much less reason to retaliate for what his partner might disclose when he experiences the therapist as accepting of his story as well as hers.

EMOTIONS

Clients who have come to talk to us against their will are emotionally upset. This upset must be acknowledged immediately and accepted with empathy. To give a message of "this is different," the therapist in general must patiently draw clients out in terms of their feelings about their situation. This is one occasion on which venting of feelings should be considered useful rather than theoretically inconsistent. When venting is followed by questions about how the therapist can be most helpful and how the clients want to use the time they have to spend in therapy, it provides the best possible groundwork for a cooperative rather than an adversarial relationship. Moreover, as discussed in Chapter 4, the opportunity to drain off anger or frustration may clear the way for solutions.

USE OF TECHNIQUES

Capricious use of techniques can hinder the development and maintenance of a good working relationship. Imagine asking about exceptions when a client is complaining about having had to stand in the rain to wait for the bus to bring him to therapy, which he thinks is unnecessary in the first place!

Imagine asking a miracle question of a mother whose child was removed from her home because of physical abuse who is complaining that she has completed parenting classes and made many changes but they never seem good enough for the social worker who visits her home!

These questions trivialize the client's feelings at the time. I have found premature use of techniques particularly irritating to involuntary clients. It seems to make them even more defensive and can thereby reinforce their aversion to therapy.

A good rule of thumb is to postpone the use of techniques until clients are ready to clarify what they think is helpful to talk about. Until then, the answers to the well-known solution-focused questions are self-evident.

THE TREATMENT SYSTEM

When clients have been mandated to therapy as part of a judgment, or as a diversion from sentencing, therapists often do not have much choice about working with them. We do not have the option of sending them away until they are ready to engage in treatment unless that is a condition we are able to establish for our own practice. We also automatically become part of a system that has taken control of the clients' life and we must understand that all those who comprise that system can only benefit the client ultimately if their efforts are coordinated.

Take Sally, a solution-focused therapist, who was an employee of a family service agency that had a rehabilitation program for drug addicts. Stan, a 32-year-old man who was on probation for possession and sale of marijuana, had been mandated to treatment in this program as part of his sentence. Stan lived with his girlfriend, Nancy, and her 10-year-old son, Al. Al was in a class for emotionally disturbed children at school and enrolled in a community-sponsored program that provided therapy for him and the family. Sally became part of a system of legal and mental health personnel involved with Stan that included the judge who sentenced Stan, Stan's probation officer, Stan's psychiatrist who was prescribing medicine for depression, a social worker from Al's program who visited the home periodically, and Al's family therapist with whom Stan met every 2 weeks along with Nancy and Al. Sally should be prepared to think beyond using her solution-focused skills with Stan. She would probably be much more helpful to him if she considered herself part of a treatment system. Moreover, she, too, was bound by the court order. Her therapy would have more of an impact if she found out what approach other mental health professionals and the social worker were taking with Stan and his family. Were they discussing his use of marijuana as addiction or disease while she was working on small steps to increase motivation to gradually reduce the frequency of smoking? If so, Stan would get confused messages and probably relapse quickly. Finally, it would benefit Sally to be aware of the judicial system's expectations for her work with Stan and her own agency's expectations. Agencies may sometimes have different ideas from therapists about the direction a case should take based on their relationship with other systems in the community.

A guiding concept for such a complicated process is clinical case management (Bachrach, 1989; Frankel & Gelman, 1998; Kanter, 1989; Moxley, 1989; Raiff & Shore, 1993) that is grounded in systemic thinking. Kanter (1989) defines clinical case management as "a modality of mental health practice" (p. 361) not merely an administrative system of coordinating services. Raiff and Shore (1993) see clinical case management as "more focused on the changes, options, and pacing of relationships" than general case management. They believe "it builds on an infrastructure of the generic skills of assessment, planning, linking, monitoring and advocacy and weds this to client engagement, consultation, and collaboration [with] other treating clinicians, individual psychotherapy, psychoeducation, and crisis intervention" (p. 85).

Like general case management, clinical case management assumes interventions will have to take place on the "micro level" (personal/interpersonal areas), "mezzo level" institutional/organization/ community issues), and "macro level" (social policy/governmental/ cultural issues) (Frankel & Gelman, 1998, p. 12). This manner of conceptualizing treatment helps maintain a perspective on the process of the system and avoids getting stuck on content (what is wrong with the identified client).

Quite clearly, we are talking about complex situations made up of variables that may diverge more than they converge. There may be a protocol to follow when child abuse is uncovered, but no case is alike when it comes to the particulars, like family relationships, involvement of other agencies, and economic and cultural factors (Alizur, 1996). Figure 3 is a systemic schema for mapping and tracking all the participants in a case and their goals. It is designed to coordinate the solution-focused therapist's work with that of others and to prevent clients from getting conflicting messages.

From a solution-focused perspective, coordinating treatment means focusing on process and communicating about content. Harlene Anderson says, "The key to successful cooperation is to talk to the other professionals in the language of their belief system" (quoted in Wynn, McDaniel, & Weber, 1986, p. 298). Another way to think about this is that one must treat members of the system like clients.

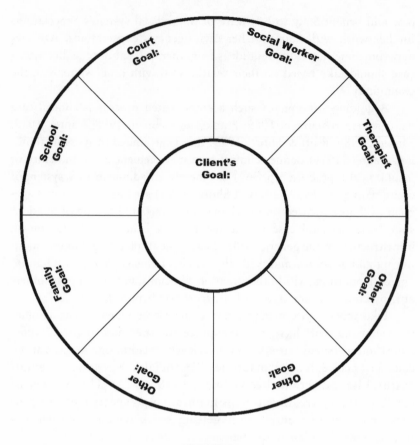

FIGURE 3

CASE EXAMPLE: CONSULTATION WITH BEA

Bea, a solution-focused family therapist and member of the Treatment Foster Care division of a family agency, came to consult about the McGee family. The identified patient was Susi, age 9, who had been in treatment foster care for 2 years. Prior to foster care Susi had had two brief hospitalizations and a 3-month stay in a residential treatment center to help her deal with her temper tantrums, firesetting, and generally unmanageable behavior at home and at school. Her mother, Lee, drank heavily prior to Susi's placement, but was in recovery for the past 1½ years.

Lee had been living with Tom for 6 years. He was also a recovering alcoholic for the past year. Before the couple stopped drinking, Tom had battered Lee several times to the point that she needed medical help. Lee never reported him to the police because she blamed herself for the fights. She suffered from recurrent depression that caused her to withdraw from Tom and culminated in suicidal ideations or gestures that led to hospitalizations. Lee decided to break up with Tom but never stuck to her decision for more than a month or two.

Lee had another child, 14-year-old David, who was a quiet boy with some learning disabilities. He had a different father than Susi.

The agency Bea worked for wanted Susi reunited with her family as soon as possible because the social worker representing the purchasing agent was putting pressure on them to do so. Susi had been doing very well in the foster home and at school for 6 months. However, her behavior in her own home remained unpredictable. It seemed to depend on Lee's emotional state.

Below are the questions the consultant asked Bea to consider. These questions reflect a solution-focused approach.

1. Who is the identified patient and what does he or she want?
   Answer: Susi is the identified patient. She wants to live with her mother, Tom, and David.
2. Who else is involved in this case and what do they want?
   Answer:
   a. The family—Lee, Tom, and David. They want Susi to come home.
   b. The foster parents. They want Susi to stay with them. They even want to adopt her.
   c. Susi's therapist. She wants her to stay in the foster home. There was no psychiatrist involved since Susi was no longer on medication.
   d. The social worker. She wants Susi to go home.
   e. The school. There was no concern about where Susi lives as long as she continues to behave while in school.
   f. Bea's agency. Bea had gotten the message that she should try to facilitate Susi's return home, if at all possible.
   g. Bea. She wants to help Susi and the family to achieve their goals, but in concert with her colleagues, if possible. She also wants to satisfy her employer.

When different parts of the system have such opposing goals, a solution that satisfies everyone is unlikely. Therefore, the consultant suggested looking at what is working for Susi and her family as a possible linkage.

3. What is working?

Answer: Susi has been doing well in the foster home and at school for 6 months. Mom and Tom have not been drinking for over a year and there is no more physical abuse. Mom has a good relationship with her therapist and psychiatrist. David is not a problem.

4. How can this positive information be reinforced so Susi can return home and behave?

Answer: Since Susi's behavior appeared to be linked with her

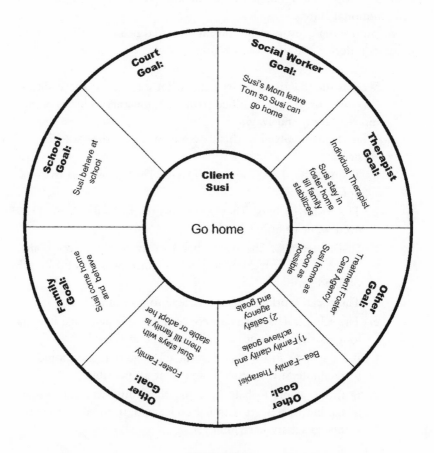

FIGURE 4

mother's depressions, and since the depressions only occurred when Lee was living with Tom, it made sense that Lee end her relationship with Tom. But that had not happened in the past and that was not the family's stated goal.

The consultant then suggested that Bea consider the case from the mother's perspective. In trying to answer the aforementioned four questions about Lee that were posed about Susi, Bea realized that she needed to gather more information. At the next consultation she was able to provide the following information:

1. Who is the client and what does he/she want?
   Answer: Lee is the client. She wants to live with Tom and her children. She does not want to have to choose between Tom and Susi.
2. Who else is involved in the case and what do they want?
   a. Tom. He wants to live with Lee and her children without conflict. He was hoping Lee's depressive episodes would end because of the negative effect they have on their relationship.
   b. Lee's psychiatrist. He feels strongly that Lee must end her relationship with Tom. He has been trying to convince her of the advantages of this for 2 years.
   c. Lee's therapist. She works in tandem with the psychiatrist and has also been urging Lee to leave Tom.
   d. The social worker. She is also convinced that the solution to this situation is for Lee to leave Tom.
   e. Bea. She wants to help the family to achieve their goal. She also wants to coordinate her work with the other professionals and satisfy her agency's goal.
3. What is working?
   Answer: There are times when Lee is not depressed. At those times she can handle Susi. Lee and Tom's relationship has positive aspects. Bea believes that Lee and Tom are very attracted to each other and truly care for each other in spite of their fighting. They have some common goals, including sobriety, and support each other in many ways. They managed the little money they have well.
4. How can these positives be reinforced to make a difference in Lee's depression?
   Answer: While gathering information Bea learned that for a

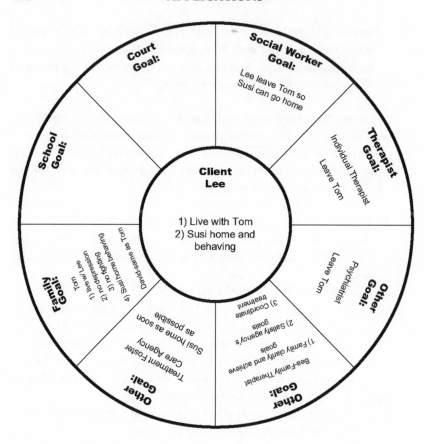

FIGURE 5

number of years now Lee had been feeling torn between what she thought she wanted for her life—to stay with Tom—and what her psychiatrist and therapist thought best for her—to leave him. Since Lee thinks highly of both her health care providers, this dilemma would become so unbearable at times that she contemplated suicide. During hospitalizations she would become increasingly certain that she must leave Tom and would act on that when she was discharged. But after some time she missed him, and invited him to come back home. Lee was always very ashamed when she took Tom back because she felt she disappointed her therapist and psychiatrist. Gradually this would lead to depression and the cycle repeated. Tom described that he gets very upset when Lee starts withdrawing from him. They begin to fight and Susi becomes noticeably harder to manage. Tom reacts to Susi by getting stricter and Lee compensates by giving in more.

It was now evident that a different treatment plan was called for to resolve this situation. One option was to see whether it would make a difference for the family if Lee and Tom made some changes in their relationship. Couple therapy had never been suggested because the therapist and psychiatrist viewed the case from a psychodynamic perspective and were working toward strengthening Lee's ego so she could leave Tom. Given these goals, Bea wondered how she could get the necessary support from the other professionals for a referral for couple treatment for Lee and Tom.

With the help of the consultant Bea developed an outline for a conversation with other professionals based on utilizing their point of view, or cooperating with it.

"I am calling to ask how you think Lee is doing because we have to make some decisions about Susi. I know Lee and Susi seem to do better when Tom is not in the home but she doesn't seem to have enough ego strength to leave him permanently. On a scale from 0 to 10, with 10 being excellent and 0 the worst if can be, at what point would you rate Lee's ego strength now, compared to when you started working with her? [Chances are that there would be report of some progress.] Yes, I have seen a little progress, too, and I think her work with you is really paying off. The meds seem to have stabilized her and the alcohol recovery continues to go well. I'm getting some pressure to move her back home. What do you think about that? [The other professionals will probably feel Susi needs to remain in the foster home. Bea will then try to solicit their support for a different strategy to strengthen Lee's ego, and stabilize Susi's behavior in Lee's home.] In talking with Lee, I have always been struck with the fact that she and Tom have a lot of good things going in their relationship in spite of the bad. His recovery seems to be going well, too. Has she shared any of that with you, too?

"I know she has a very good relationship with you and she tries to please all the time, but at the same time we all know she is passive–aggressive. I have been doing some consulting about this case and wonder whether you would join me in considering a different approach with Lee, just as an experiment. Maybe if we tried to stop influencing Lee to leave Tom she might feel less inclined to resist it so much. It might free her up to make a different choice than just opposing us. She may also have some ideas about what she and Tom need to live together more peacefully.

"The suggestion is that everyone who works with Lee tell her, in our own way, that we have come to realize that she really wants to be with Tom because the good in the relationship seems to outweigh the bad for her. Since we understand that now, we want to try to help her and Tom work things out. We could suggest couple therapy to improve the relationship."

Bea also had to get the county social worker on board for this experiment. They had worked fairly well together in the past. In this case, however, they disagreed, and the social worker had given up on Lee and her ability to change. She had begun to threaten Lee with further court conditions such as severely restricted visits with Susi, supervised visits, and even termination of parental rights if she did not leave Tom. The therapist expected the social worker to be very much against the suggested plan. Bea and the consultant then planned to introduce the conversation with the social worker as follows:

"I know you've had it with Lee. We've all been trying hard but you were expecting more progress. We are disappointed, as well. I have recently done some consulting on this case and I wonder whether you would consider an experiment. It would include the psychiatrist and individual therapist as well. It's worth giving it just one more try—to do something different—as nothing else has worked with Lee and Tom and to get Susi home. It's a long shot, but if it works it will speed things up and you won't have to go through the messy court procedures. I'm not sure you'll agree with this, but I have seen this approach work before in stuck cases."

Naturally, there is no guarantee that this type of conversation will have the desired effect on others, but even if it does not, there is a chance that the suggestion itself could make a small change in their thinking that could lead to other changes.

However, in the case of the McGee family, the other professionals did agree to go along with Bea's suggestion. Lee and Tom attended couple therapy sessions for 6 months and toward the end Lee came to a decision on her own to end her relationship with Tom. She recognized that his expectations for attention from her were too much for her to meet. Tom came to believe and accept that Lee was unable to meet his emotional needs. After the couple separated Lee did not ask Tom to return. Susi came home and Lee was able to manage her well.

The idea that Bea, the family therapist, should take it upon herself to make an indirect intervention in the treatment system will undoubtedly raise some questions. We usually think that colleagues, much like clients, should talk openly with each other and negotiate their differences. Of course, this is always the preferred way to go, especially if all the professionals share a common theoretical orientation, but in professional relationships, as well as personal ones, hierarchical issues and other struggles often obstruct progress.

Systemic coordination requires the ability to step back and look at the interactions of all parts of the system, family as well as professionals. This is the expertise of family therapists. Many mental health professionals are schooled to view problems as residing within the identified patient. When a case is stuck and one person has expertise that the others do not have, his or her suggestion may not always be received with an open mind. Yet, he or she owes it to the clients to find a way to persuade the others to give it a try, as long as it is in a respectful manner and will not endanger anyone.

CONCLUSION

Working with involuntary clients, particularly the mandated ones, requires ecosystemic as well as solution-focused thinking. It resembles family therapy because it calls for helping parties with frequently different needs and wants to achieve a common goal. What makes it more difficult than family therapy is that there is no unifying resource (e.g., family ties) to provide a foundation for solutions. On the contrary, clients usually perceive their relationship with their helpers and the law to be an adversarial one. The solution-focused model may not always be the answer to the complex cases described here, but its focus on individual strengths and interactional process gives it a better than average chance for avoiding impasse or failure.

11

Long-Term Cases

What is the meaning of the phrase "long-term case"? It suggests that there are some distinctions to be made before the start of treatment, or at the beginning of it, that categorize a case as either short or long term. This way of thinking is not consistent with solution-focused theory and practice. While the Mental Research Institute model and SFT are known to be brief models, "brief" in that sense is a by-product of their focused approach, not of the intent to work as quickly as possible. The primary goal is effective problem resolution. In fact, prejudgments about the potential length of a case hinders cooperation with clients and belies the assumption that *therapists cannot change clients; clients can only change themselves.*

For example, it is not illogical to think that the case of a client who just lost his leg in an accident and can no longer work at his customary job will be "long term." Under those circumstances, most people might need a lot of therapeutic support over a considerable amount of time while grieving their losses. Yet, there are people who value helping themselves, above all. For them, extended therapy only compounds their problem by pointing to the loss of their independence. All they may need is an understanding ear, compliments about how well they are coping, and reminders about past coping skills that they can use now and in the future.

On the other hand, when a single mother states her goal at the beginning of therapy as "I want my 3-year-old son to sleep in his own bed," one might think this problem could result in a "short-term" case.

However, that goal may be a complaint (content) that reflects a process in the mother's life that affects much more than her child's sleeping habits (e.g., her general lack of assertiveness). How brief the case will be depends on whether a solution to the stated problem (content) satisfies the client—whether he or she presents other problems dealing with the process—and on his or her ability and readiness to change.

There are situations in which the length of cases is determined by the referral source, such as some managed care cases or court-referred ones. Managed care companies often predetermine treatment to last no more than 6 or 10 sessions, while judges can mandate treatment for as long as a year or more. Either prescription can lead to inadequate service, as the duration of a case must be determined based on clients' needs not on a particular time frame. The best way to handle these situations is to discuss them with the clients. What will be most helpful if only six sessions are authorized? What is best if goals are reached before the 12 months of mandated treatment has elapsed? Clients need to know that they must fulfill their obligation but that they can help determine the options.

A solution-focused case may span months or years but differs from what is traditionally thought of as long-term therapy because it consists of an ebb and flow of contact, depending on the client's needs, rather than a period of uninterrupted weekly or bimonthly appointments. Each episode of treatment has its own goal that contributes to an overall goal.

For example, consider the case of a man who is taking care of his wife who is deteriorating from multiple sclerosis. He is sent for therapy by his physician because of stress-related somatic symptoms. However, the client says what he wants from coming to therapy is to be more patient with his wife. Treatment could be very short if the client identifies what is different when he is more patient (say when allows himself a little time away from her) and does more of that. A few visits is all the help he may ever need.

On the other hand, he may not know what makes the difference, or he may know but not do more about it. Then this first phase of treatment may last for several months until the client achieves his goal. After that, there may be less contact, or none, until the client feels he has a problem again. The wife may have been placed in a nursing home meanwhile. The client feels he needs respite from daily visits but does not know how to tell her. Again the goal has to be clarified and the client may find a solution quickly or slowly. What defines cases such as this as "brief therapy" is the underlying philosophy of helping clients use their own strengths and remain as self-reliant as possible.

Before looking at typical situations that need therapist–client contact over prolonged periods, it might be useful to consider how we determine when a case is ready to be terminated in the first place.

TERMINATION: THE CLIENT'S PROBLEM

It has been my experience that when brief therapy is going well, therapists and clients come to the realization that it is time to stop meeting at almost the same time. At that point, clients may feel they have nothing to talk about, and therapists may feel they have asked once too often what clients will do to prevent the problems in the future or to fix it if it should occur again. There are situations, however, when termination is not that clear.

The most obvious one is when clients admit that they have achieved their goal but are afraid to terminate because they fear relapse. When this becomes evident, either because the client says so directly or because he or she begins presenting new problems we believe he or she has the capacity to solve, there is one more task to be accomplished. The client must develop the confidence to stop talking with us.

When the anxiety is expressed overtly, a useful thing to do is to normalize it and offer another appointment for a month hence, with the suggestion that it may be canceled if it is no longer needed.

When the fear of termination is expressed by means of a new problem, we must first determine whether or not this problem is related to the process the client just dealt with successfully. Successful resolution of one problem may have given a client the courage to face a totally different one. On the other hand, if the client had just achieved a successful way of dealing with anger, and he or she presented a new problem dealing with anger, we could refer the client back to the skills he or she had just acquired. I once had a client who was capable of helping herself, but after two termination sessions she found an excuse to call for another appointment. I finally told her that the next time she called I would only see her if she could first tell me that she had successfully resolved two problems in the meantime. She said, "You just don't want to see me anymore." I answered, "No. I just want you to have the confidence that you can help yourself. As long as you keep seeing me you won't have that confidence."

TERMINATION: THE THERAPIST'S PROBLEM

Therapists usually determine whether therapy is over by whether clients feel they have achieved what they came for. If they have not, the therapist has to start reclarifying with the clients what they want and build from there.

However, consulting with solution-focused therapists has made me aware of the fact that some therapists believe a case is stuck when, in fact, it was over a long time ago. The following case is a typical example.

CASE EXAMPLE: CONSULTATION WITH JOE

Joe asked for consultation about a case that he had been seeing continually for a year and a half. He felt things had improved overall but that something was missing that prevented the client from fully achieving her goal.

When Joe first began seeing Mandy, a 28-year-old, single woman, she was unemployed. She had a history of trying different types of jobs and leaving them because they did not satisfy her. She was also in a dating relationship with a man whom she felt used by. Mandy had presented with symptoms of depression and said she did not know who she is and what she wants from life. When Joe had asked her how she would know she did not have to come anymore she said she would be working in a job she liked, would feel enjoyment in life at least 80% of the time, and would be in a relationship in which she felt valued.

Mandy had chosen to focus on her job situation first. Within 6 months (10 sessions) she was working as a hostess in a restaurant chain and liking it. After the first 10 sessions Mandy reported that the job improved her enjoyment of life from 25 to 50%.

Shortly thereafter she chose to end her relationship. She had made some more attempts to get her needs met by her boyfriend but when he did not respond she decided she would rather be lonely than be treated badly.

During the next 5 months she grieved the relationship in therapy but also began to define what her expectations were for a future one. When she began to date another man who was more attentive to her, she used therapy to guide her in making choices for herself in relation to this man. By the time Mandy had been seeing Joe for a year, her rating of her satisfaction with life fluctuated between 75% and 80%, except when she experienced some stress at work or in the relationship. Then it could dip to 50 or 60% for short periods.

By the time of the consultation, Mandy was the manager of a branch of the restaurant chain for which she had started working after she started therapy. Her relationship with her new boyfriend was progressing well due to their ability to discuss differences and to work them out.

Joe described the client as an attractive young woman who had become very dependent on his reassurance. He recognized how well she was doing but was concerned because Mandy did not feel sure enough of herself yet and her rate of satisfaction with life was not steady at 80%. The consultation centered on the following points:

Job Situation

CONSULTANT: The client seems to be set in a career and liking it. What is the nature of the stress she is experiencing at work and do you think she is capable of handling it?

JOE: Her problems are nothing out of the ordinary for a management position. She usually discusses her way of handling them with me and she has become very capable.

CONSULTANT: So she uses good judgment?

JOE: Yes, but she is not confident that it is good judgment.

CONSULTANT: On a scale of 1 to 10, with 10 being as confident as anyone can get, how confident are you that she can handle the problems?

JOE: Eight . . . 9 . . .

CONSULTANT: And how confident do you think Mandy is?

JOE: Well, at times she is seems like a 10, but when things go wrong she dips to a 2 or 3. Hmm . . . I guess she tends to overreact anyway . . . that's her style.

At this point Joe recognized that he was overreacting to Mandy's overreactions and that he needed to respond to her with more confidence in her own resources when she came for help with problems.

Relationship

Joe was also concerned about the stability of Mandy's relationship because her boyfriend had not asked her to move in with him yet. The consultant wondered whether there were signs that Mandy was being used again, and Joe said there did not seem to be any. The young man appeared to be sincere and caring but not ready for a full commitment until he finished his master's degree in 6 months.

CONSULTANT: What do you think Mandy needs in terms of the relationship?

JOE: Pretty much what she is getting. I just don't want her to get hurt again.

CONSULTANT: From what you said, the chances seem pretty slim.

JOE: I think so.

CONSULTANT: And if he did hurt her, how do you think she would handle it compared to when you first met her?

JOE: Much better. Her work is fulfilling and she has made more friends.

Again, Joe recognized that he was being overprotective.

Enjoyment of Life

Mandy was not reporting 75% enjoyment of life on a steady basis.

CONSULTANT: What would happen if she did?

JOE: It would be time to terminate.

CONSULTANT: Do you think the client wants to terminate?

JOE: No, I think she's afraid she can't manage.

CONSULTANT: How do you feel about terminating her?

Joe now realized that he was dealing with some separation problems from Mandy as well, and that he had been instrumental in her dependence on therapy.

The consultant wondered what Joe would do at this point if Mandy had to move to another city in a month, or her insurance benefits ran out? Joe knew that he had to respond less to Mandy's uncertainty and support her strengths more. To accomplish this goal Joe would have to normalize the work stresses and the relationship issues and refer Mandy back to times when she handled similar problems successfully. Joe realized he had yet to work with Mandy on how to handle certain situations in the future. He thought that he would handle termination gently over the period of a few sessions with the assurance that the door would always be open if Mandy needed to come back for a "booster shot."

Joe also had to recognize that he would have to deal with the loss of his relationship with Mandy and put it in proper perspective. He had the courage to admit that perhaps he had not considered termination sooner because Mandy is an attractive young woman whose company and admiration he enjoyed. It is not unusual that when therapists become attached to clients for reasons of their own, brief therapy can turn into long-term therapy.

THERAPIST'S SELF-EVALUATION
FOR TERMINATION

One of the qualities of SFT and other models that look to the clients to define what they want from therapy is that they have the ability to keep us honest. If we truly accept what clients are saying about what they want from therapy and what is changing for them, we will not keep seeing them longer than necessary. The sooner clients can feel they do not need therapy anymore, the stronger and more competent they will feel.

The most prevalent cause for short-term cases to become long-term cases is that therapists forget that *clients have the strengths and resources to help themselves.* Therapists can be perfectionistic or overprotective at times and continue to see clients longer than necessary. Their intention is to make sure the clients are all right and to reinforce changes while the message to the client is "I don't trust that you can be all right without me."

The ideal termination occurs when clients report a solution, the therapist gives them an appointment for a month later, the solution is still reported to be working, and clients and therapist shake hands and say good-bye. To have as many ideal terminations as possible, and to keep cases as brief as possible, frank self-examination about our feelings toward clients is a must. We must ask ourselves, "Am I continuing to see him because he is asking me to, and I like to please people? Is she interesting or a sexually attractive person whom I enjoy being around? Does he have authorization for 10 sessions and although his problem was resolved in 6 sessions the income from a few sessions benefits me and will not harm him? Do I want her to achieve some goals I think will benefit her but they have not specified?"

Of course, we also have to face the times we may terminate clients hastily because we do not like them, feel unsuccessful with them, or even fear them.

CLIENTS WITH CHRONIC PROBLEMS

Clients with chronic physical or emotional problems vary in their ability to function independently. Some may work and support themselves financially while others depend on disability insurance. They may seek psychotherapy on their own or be referred by a helping professional.

One of the many burdens of a chronic condition is the label it imparts. Such a health problem can result in a negative self-image or prejudice on the part of others. It affects expectations and therefore potential productivity. The strength-based philosophy girding SFT is a helpful approach in these cases because of its assumption that *every client is unique* and, therefore, unique in his or her possibilities for change.

I have personally experienced a situation in which a client who had been diagnosed as chronically depressed 9 years earlier made a total recovery and lifestyle change when reevaluated and treated by a solution-focused therapist who recognized his strengths. This case is an exception but evidence, nevertheless, that we must keep an open mind with every client with whom we work.

CASE EXAMPLE: VIRGINIA

The case of Virginia is an example of how labels can obscure strengths and the importance of the therapist–client relationship in longer cases (Kreider, 1998). Virginia was a 42-year old woman on social security disability who was referred by her social worker for anger management. She was grossly overweight, had had surgery for a cleft palate, and walked poorly because of a club foot. Her biological mother died when Virginia was 3. Her father remarried 2 years later. He and her stepmother terminated their parental rights when Virginia was 16 because of their inability to control her aggressive behavior. She never had contact with them again. She became a ward of the state and lived in foster homes until age 17, at which time she was placed in a hospital for the chronically mentally ill. Her records indicated a variety of diagnoses including schizophrenia, chronic depression, and borderline personality disorder with psychotic episodes. The hospital had kept her under heavy sedation to contain her behavior. A stroke of luck led to her deinstitutionalization 11 years later. A new psychiatric resident on her ward became interested in Virginia's case and was able to convince his supervisors to take her off all the medications and switch her to lithium and a tranquilizer. The results were dramatic enough to allow Virginia to live independently with social service support. When I first met Virginia she was living with a man whom she had met several years ago. Her only other contact was with a foster mother who lived in another part of the state.

Virginia's social worker had described her as a difficult client who could not get along with people and who had been fired by her last therapist. Our first session suggested to me that Virginia was very anxious because she avoided eye contact and spouted an uninterruptable stream of anger about everything in her life.

Virginia and I had a relationship that lasted 12 years. Six of those years consisted of the following phases of treatment:

1. The first 2 months Virginia came irregularly and was basically uncooperative. She refused to respond to any solution talk. Because *nothing is all negative* and *brief therapy goes slowly* I decided to wait and concentrate on the emotional climate. Virginia had four cats she called her "babies" of whom she spoke tenderly. I frequently inquired about the cats.

Beginning with the third month Virginia started to come regularly every week and began to share some of her history. She still refused to talk about goals.

2. Virginia was transported to sessions by a service provided by social services. About 6 months after we started meeting, her social worker called and said that the company that ran the vans was threatening to refuse transporting her because she was verbally abusive to the drivers.

I raised this in our session but Virginia denied any responsibility. When I expressed regret that this would keep us from meeting in the future she first ignored me but eventually admitted that it would be better if she had someone to talk to, especially someone who did not tell her what to do. I accepted her anger at the drivers as legitimate and questioned her about it. It turned out that she insulted the drivers because she did not think they were sensitive enough when handling some of the disabled patients on the van.

THERAPIST: What do you think you can do other than getting angry at the driver when you feel anxious that someone might get hurt or be uncomfortable?

VIRGINIA: Keep my mouth shut.

THERAPIST: But that's hard! Especially when you are concerned.

VIRGINIA: You bet! They don't keep theirs shut at all.

THERAPIST: Are there times when you see something that concerns you and you do something other than get angry at the driver?

VIRGINIA: Like what?

THERAPIST: I don't know. What other things do you do on the van ride when you get upset?

VIRGINIA: Shut up or scream!

THERAPIST: What else could you do?

VIRGINIA: Beats me.

THERAPIST: I've heard people say that when they are in a situation that concerns them they just ask the person in charge whether they are aware that there might be some danger.

VIRGINIA: They don't want me to open my mouth period.

THERAPIST: Is that something you want to do . . . not open your mouth?

VIRGINIA: Hmm . . . I can't do that when I'm angry.

THERAPIST: Would you like to try some things that could help?

VIRGINIA: Yeah! But . . . it would take a miracle.

I built on her use of the word "miracle" to ask a miracle question. She could not answer at first but the question reminded her of an exception: Sometimes when she thought hard about something else she was able to control herself. What might she want to think about on the van? She said her cats. She would try to say their names over and over again when she felt angry.

Virginia tried for a week but had another outburst that resulted in the cancellation of her rides. This fueled her rage again, and I spent quite a bit of time on the phone listening to her and complimenting her for having attempted to control her temper in the first place. I then offered to call the van company and advocate for her. She reluctantly agreed. Virginia was given another chance and there were no further complaints. Subsequently, I complimented Virginia every time we met on her ability to exercise such control and we discussed in detail how she was doing it. In addition to saying her cats' names she had began to count red cars and observe other things outside the van.

3. After this incident Virginia became more focused. She said she wanted to work on being less frustrated. Which frustration in her life did she want to work on first? Her relationship with her boyfriend, Sam. What aspects of that relationship frustrated her? *A small change can lead to bigger changes.* His not answering her when she talked to him. It was difficult for Virginia to stick to this specific complaint about Sam but the process of her nagging and his withdrawing seemed to improve. Sam joined us for some of the sessions. I used solution-focused questions and built on what was working for them as a couple. We talked a lot about their feelings and I reinforced the positives in their relationship repeatedly. On a scale on which 1 represented a very bad relationship and 10 represented the best they could imagine, they both reported a change from 3 to 7.

4. Winter was approaching and I had been seeing Virginia almost weekly for close to a year. Her social worker was reporting that she was more relaxed and in control, so I suggested that we begin to meet every other week. I had to do this carefully and not make it seem like a rejection. Virginia had begun to enjoy our weekly meetings and I used her empathy for people with disabilities to say that by coming less frequently she would be making room for someone else who needed help. I offered her phone contact between sessions in case she needed it. She responded well to this and only rarely called.

5. Five months later one of Virginia's cats was run over. This loss triggered other losses in her life, such as the death of her biological mother and the loss of contact with the psychiatrist who rescued her. For about 6 months we resumed weekly sessions to support her alternate sadness and rage which also had repercussions in her relationship with Sam.

6. When things stabilized again we gradually reduced the frequency of sessions and dealt with occasional minor crises over the phone. During those phone calls it was enough to let her vent and then to ask her what she needed to calm down in a manner that would make her feel good about herself.

During the next 2 years I saw Virginia when there was a crisis—for example, when she fought with her landlord over some repairs for which she believed he had unjustly held her and Sam responsible. She eventually resolved this situation by drawing on what she had learned from dealing with the van drivers and rehearsing new, nonconfrontive ways of negotiating.

7. Virginia came in for the last interlude of sessions 6 years after we first met. Sam had lost his job and was very depressed. She reacted with anger and frustration. We had weekly visits again and the couple eventually decided to move closer to her foster mother who was beginning to have health problems.

Saying good-bye to Virginia was not easy for me either. Over the years I had begun to appreciate the woman who hid behind a frequently angry façade: this kind, honest, and intelligent person with an amazing amount of resilience. My respect for her was to grow even more, however.

8. Virginia kept in touch occasionally after she moved. She had connected with a therapist and psychiatrist at her new location but she still called occasionally, and visited once, a few years later. There were always cards at Christmas and Easter. I was informed when any of the cats died or a new one was acquired.

Three years later the calls increased because Sam was diagnosed as having stomach cancer. Virginia nursed Sam at home for a whole year. They were married 2 months before he died. She was an incredibly patient, giving nurse. As his time grew short, they planned Sam's funeral together, including what he would wear in the casket. After Sam died I heard from Virginia less frequently for a while.

Then, about 8 months later I received an audiotape in the mail that Virginia had made in the middle of the night. She was experiencing terrible grief and could not sleep. She asked me to reply on the tape and send it back. We exchanged tapes four or five times and Virginia gradually began to feel better. Her social worker was looking for some volunteer work for her to do in the community that would not tax her too much physically or emotionally. The last time I heard from Virginia she was moving again and then we lost contact.

This is long-term, or supportive, SFT. It can result in considerable changes, depending on the innate capacity of the particular client. It is guided by the basic assumptions but it often extends beyond the therapy room, much like casework.

CASE EXAMPLE: THE MAN WHO HEARD VOICES[1]

SFT is suitable for clients who have been hearing voices all their life. It offers a relationship with a therapist who accepts, rather than challenges, their point of view, thereby reducing anxiety. This relationship can stabilize and lead to a greater sense of personal control and agency for clients.

Fred was a 45-year-old white male on social security disability who had been in the mental health system for 25 years. He lived alone and worked part time delivering interoffice mail at a large corporation. He first heard voices when he started college, and he dropped out shortly thereafter. He was referred by his social worker who expressed concern that Fred's use of alcohol was getting out of hand. He was under the care of a psychiatrist who dispensed and monitored his medications.

THERAPIST: Could you tell me what is your understanding of why you are here?

FRED: My caseworker said I should come in. He gets worried sometimes when he comes to my house and sees all the beer bottles around.

THERAPIST: What is it about all the beer bottles that makes him worry about you?

FRED: He thinks I am drinking too much. Maybe I am sometimes, but if you had to go through what I go through you would be drinking, too. Do you drink?

THERAPIST: Never at work. (*Fred laughs.*) Your caseworker must really care about you if he worries so much. Have you two been working together long?

FRED: Oh yeah, he comes over twice a week. He brings me shopping. He helps me write bills. It really makes a difference. Years ago when I was in the hospital I never thought I'd get out, you know, free again. Being in the program helps a lot.

THERAPIST: What worries you about the drinking?

FRED: Nothing much worries me. I do spend too much money but sometimes it is the only thing to do. You know, often I'll go into a bar

---

[1]This case description was provided by Brett Brasher of the Mental Health Center of Dane County, Wisconsin. It is an example of the type of case he treats frequently.

and people will look at me sort of funny. But, after a while, after I have a few beers, I am just like everyone else.

THERAPIST: But your caseworker is worried, isn't he?

FRED: Well, sometimes it's the only way.

THERAPIST: The only way?

FRED: (*Tears.*) Yeah!

THERAPIST: The only way to handle what goes on inside your head?

FRED: Yes, that's it! When I have enough to drink things get quiet, real quiet. When they are quiet I am able to think. I am able to do things. I don't hear the demons.

The therapist learned that drinking helped quiet the client's voices. Because this is a valuable coping mechanism for the client it cannot be replaced until he finds a more suitable one. Therefore, the therapist chose to go slowly and to concentrate on establishing a trusting relationship first. For a few weeks he did not urge the client to stop drinking but just showed interest in him and his life. The client began to let him into his world.

FRED: Oh God, it's funny. I say oh God, because that is what helps. I listen to God. It used to be everything that I heard in my head was the devil, demons. I had two demons—one telling me to hurt myself, the other telling me so many things you wouldn't want to hear. Now, I try to listen to God. And, as I listen to God it helps with the struggle with the temptations of the devil. God tells me not to worry about the devil. There are times I don't hear any voices. This happens generally when I work.

THERAPIST: What do you do to make that happen? [Presupposed client control.]

FRED: The first thing is I let them know that I won't listen to them when I work. Between the hours of 12 and 3 is my time. Nights are hard. I go home about 6:30 and sit in my chair and smoke cigarettes and let them come. Sometimes it takes so much energy it's hard to sleep.

THERAPIST: When things start getting better what do you suppose will be the first thing you notice?

FRED: I will have more strength. I'll have more energy and be more interesting; maybe I'll even start talking with people a bit more.

THERAPIST: Are there times when that happens already?

FRED: Sometimes, but not enough.

THERAPIST: If you would be giving advice to someone who also hears voices like you, what would you say?

FRED: I'd tell them that they need to live a life that is as stress free as possible. If you get a life with no stress and keep it that way for a long time you have a better change of surviving.

THERAPIST: Anything else?

FRED: Watch what you eat. Some foods scare demons. If you eat Moroccan or Basmati rice it tends to help.

As Brett Brasher learned more about the client's unique resources he started to make attempts to reinforce them for the future. He recommends an open-ended approach to treatment with this type of client. The experience has been going on for many years; therefore, the notion of change, though desired, it also frightening. Questions about how he will know he does not have to come anymore can evoke vision of being without support and are therefore not recommended. Progress must be handled tentatively and slowly.

This dialogue took place a couple of months into treatment.

THERAPIST: Would you say you are handling things a little bit better now than when we first started to meet?

FRED: Oh, yeah, a lot better. Last night I sat around for an hour and I was bored.

THERAPIST: Bored?

FRED: Yes, bored. I love to feel a sense of boredom. You know, it's a peaceful time. When I am bored I know there is nothing coming in. I can just be.

THERAPIST: That does sound peaceful.

FRED: I try to handle psychosis with patience and bravery. Patience and bravery will go a long way to defeat the demons.

THERAPIST: [Reassured client that he would be part of his future.] What do you need to know so that 6 months from now when we talk about this you will be feeling OK about yourself?

FRED: I need to know God's with me. You know God says that true schizophrenics have a hole in the soul. Talking with God can rescue me. And I know that even though I have been through this miserable stuff I am cultivating a good soul.

THERAPIST: As you are cultivating are you also planting?

FRED: Well, going to church scares the demons.

THERAPIST: [Followed the client's thinking rather than pursuing his own thought about planting.] When you are in church, what do you do to get a sense of serenity?

FRED: Being in church lets the demons know that I am not afraid. When in doubt, be brave. Being brave can defeat a lot of demons. Demons aren't that smart. I do have trouble later on. You know, especially in the evenings when my psychic energy lets down its defenses.

Brett Brasher also cautions against seeing clients who hear voices too frequently. Though they need ongoing support, it can be counterproductive for them to focus on the details of their life too much. He often invites clients to determine how many visits a month are most comfortable for them. This client chose to come about once a month. After about 4 months he announced that he had decided to give up drinking.

FRED: I have been sober now for 3 weeks. I decided that it didn't make much sense to come in and see you and still be drinking. What I also decided is God feels that I need to have my wits about me.

THERAPIST: Has that made a difference for you? Quitting drinking and all?

FRED: Yeah. I do find I am drinking more coffee and smoking more cigarettes. You know that when I smoke cigarettes things are quiet for a while?

The client was finding his own substitutes for drinking. He shared that inhaling a cigarette allowed him to concentrate on his breathing rather than on his brain. He also shared that he has gotten a cell phone and when the voices get too loud he takes out the phone and starts talking on it.

FRED: I look like a yuppie (*laughing*).

THERAPIST: What else helps you?

FRED: Talking with you, and I got some friends. Sometimes we get together and talk about what is going on. That's hard though. It's better just to play guitar.

THERAPIST: How did the voices react when you talked to other people about them?

FRED: Oh, they don't like it. They start getting loud and I pray. And when I do that I get the strength to break the silence.

THERAPIST: What happens when you don't listen to what the voices suggest?

FRED: Oh, they get mad. But, what I am realizing is that the virtue of fighting these demons allow for a major spiritual transformation. The illness is a change for me to get closer to God. This is my salvation. I owe God a lot. I want to pay him back. I know I owe him a lot, but I don't know where to send the check.

THERAPIST: I don't suppose that God has much need with money, so you don't need to send the check anywhere.

FRED: Yeah, you are right.

THERAPIST: Instead of sending a check, what might you do with some of the money you have saved by being sober? [Tried to guide client toward more coping strategies.]

FRED: Well, I am saving for a computer. Maybe then I could get on the Internet and talk to other people. When I type no one knows what I am thinking.

Change is not always smooth. This client had a major relapse during the next month during which he believed people were following him because St. Paul was trying to kill him for not going to church enough.

THERAPIST: What made you think it was St. Paul?

FRED: I just knew it. He was after me. It was horrible.

THERAPIST: That sounds horrible. Are you sure it was St. Paul?

FRED: (looking puzzled) Yes. What do you mean?

THERAPIST: Well, St. Paul is a saint of love. Why would a saint of love be trying to do things that would make you doubt his love? [Offering a reframe.]

FRED: I don't know.

As the therapist and client talked about St. Paul's mission the client started to change his idea of what his fears were.

FRED: Maybe St. Paul is trying to help me?

THERAPIST: I wonder if St. Paul, perhaps, may be trying to make you more aware and more conscious of things around you?

FRED: I'm going to think about that.

Working with clients who hear voices may well represent the most salient example of cooperating with clients and how solution-focused assumptions guide our work. It really challenges us to remember their strengths and resources, to work slowly and on small changes, and to realize that we cannot change them. The emotional climate is also important because it can provide the security these anxious, distrustful clients lack everywhere else in their lives.

Gradual attention to clients' emotions is also important. Brasher points out that people who hear voices are alienated from their own feelings and therefore have trouble reading the feelings of others. The relationship with the therapist can be a source of safe learning.

Relapses are also viewed as learning opportunities. Emphasis should be on "what is different about this episode?" This builds a chain of events toward a better future, which these clients usually do not have on their own.

ADJUSTMENT TO DISABILITY

Some people experience sudden or gradual deterioration in their physical condition that require major changes in lifestyle. The resulting loss of identity and inability to function as before requires major adjustments. For the solution-focused therapist this dilemma becomes a balancing act between helping clients grieve their losses and build a new life based on their past and potential resources.

CASE EXAMPLE: CAROL

Carol is a client who represents such an example. In the prime of life, at age 39, she suffered a spinal cord injury in an automobile accident with an uninsured driver. She was married, the mother of four children ages 8 to 15, and co-owner of a fashionable women's clothing boutique. Her husband was a commercial artist. The injury caused her to lose control of her bowels and bladder. She now had to control these functions mechanically, but this method was not foolproof and she could not avoid occasional accidents.

Carol was referred by her physician who felt Carol needed help in adjusting to her disability. Carol asked that her husband come in with her for the initial session. She explained that she had expected to be back at work by this time but was too weak and too fearful about offending others with a possible "accident." It became evident that Carol, a woman who had always been fully in control of her life, was experiencing herself as having lost control over every aspect of it. She had refused antidepressants or medications to relieve her anxiety on the ground that it would be one more way of giving up who she used to be. At the end of the session I acknowledged Carol's suffering but expressed amazement that she was doing as well as she was. I sincerely believed that given the circumstances many other people might not be making as much of an effort to resume their family and work responsibilities. I listed specific things Carol was trying to do (help children with homework, make grocery lists, keep in touch with business partner) to indicate that she did still have some control.

Several days after our first appointment Carol's husband called to say he had taken Carol to the emergency room the night before because she was experiencing extreme anxiety and flashbacks of her accident. The resident on call, who did not speak English too well, recommended hospitalization because he believed Carol to be having a psychotic episode. Carol's husband felt the resident had not understood Carol's medical condition well enough and investigated its possible connection with her present symptoms. When Carol refused to admit herself, the resident prescribed an antianxiety medication and urged her husband to take Carol to see a psychiatrist the next day.

I met with Carol and her husband on an emergency basis the next day. Carol expressed complete hopelessness. A suicide assessment indicated that she was not at risk. However, the events of the previous evening and the suggestion that she might also be losing control over her mind exacerbated her condition. The physician who managed Carol's case had been alerted and was meeting with Carol and her husband later that day to assess her medical status. It was Friday, and we worked on getting through the next 2 days before we would meet again.

To provide Carol with some structure and predictability we worked on writing down a detailed description of her schedule for the next 48 hours, hour by hour. The task was built on Carol's exceptions to anxiety and lack of control. As she began to contribute these ideas she felt more in control. The list included having soft jazz playing during the night, not being left alone in a room without her husband or one of the children, and not having to talk on the telephone to friends and relatives. I offered phone contact if needed but never received a call.

I met with Carol and her husband again on Monday and they reported a good weekend. The medical examination had not resulted in clear answers, but some tests had been taken and the dosage of one medication had been reduced because of possible side effect of increased anxiety. For about 2 months thereafter, Carol and I met on a weekly basis. Carol always insisted her husband come into the session with her. She used the time mainly to vent anger and frustration and I kept expressing empathy and reinforcing her efforts to cope.

Gradually, Carol's anger turned to sadness about the loss of her former self and she cried a lot. Carol was still frail physically. Too much emotional stress manifested itself in infections and other physical symptoms that weakened her. Therefore, her grieving had to be contained in a manner that did not overwhelm her. It was therefore suggested that Carol compartmentalize her grieving into two 20-minute periods a day. That gave her an opportunity not to give in to every wave of grief but to tell herself that she would postpone reacting to it until the designated time. Carol responded well to this suggestion because it proved to her she had some control.

After about 8 months Carol began to show signs of improvement. She was gaining more control over her hygiene problems. She cried less, was more future oriented, and began to think about the future of her career. She needed appointments less frequently.

However, as things got better for Carol, her husband and children began to release some of the stress they had had to contain for so long. Conflicts between her husband and their oldest son began to erupt, and a daughter began to act out at school. At Carol's request we had family sessions for several months to debrief the difficult events of the past and shape a future that fit the present circumstances while still considering the needs of individual family members.

During the next 2 years Carol's progress was slow and steady, though interspersed with some critical episodes that required periods of more frequent visits. From time to time her anger about her losses would resurface and she would need help keeping it separate from family, friends, and her doctors. On those occasions she needed support and permission to keep venting her anger. Although she had become strong enough to drive and live more independently, Carol had to accept that she could never function at her former pace again. This led to a painful decision to sell her part of her business and began a search for a fulfilling activity she could do from home.

Aside from listening and accepting her feelings to deal with her losses, what seemed to help Carol the most was to ask her to scale her progress since her accident, to think about what had contributed to that progress, and to ask what was needed for another small step forward. This helped Carol become more skillful at helping herself. The more confident she felt about being independent from therapy, the more control she felt, and the more control she felt, the better she functioned on a physical and emotional level.

Four years later Carol terminated provisionally with the condition that she could call any time she needed. Before that step, she had gone through another period of grief triggered by her father's death. However, when Carol recovered from that loss she rated the quality of her life an 8 on a scale of 10, with 10 being the best she could ever have expected herself to feel given her condition.

CONCLUSION

It is suggested that solution-focused therapists not think in terms of short- or long-term cases. When problems are considered to be the inner and outer perturbations that have to be adjusted in the drift through life, then classifying them hardly seems useful for clients or therapists. The solution to the survival and well-being of one person may take two sessions, whereas for another it may take the form of lifelong episodes of support and problem solving interspersed with periods of well-being. The issue is not how long the treatment lasts but what the best solution is for the particular client.

The most favorable outcome for clients who require episodic treatment is that it is guided by the assumption that *a small change can lead to bigger changes*. When each episode is handled like a separate problem that needs a solution, rather than a part of an overall disability, clients maintain hope and confidence in themselves. By the same token, when gradual loss of function is treated as the conservation of functioning as well as a continuing loss, clients can grieve as well as maintain some courage.

Treating cases over longer periods may challenge therapists who are accustomed to using the solution-focused approach to work briefly. Episodic work over a longer period usually requires more patience, at least at first. The types of clients who comes back to see us on and off for years may be so accustomed to being treated as helpless or deficient by families and helpers that they may take a long time to recognize they can be instrumental in their own solutions. Long-term relationships with clients also make professional detachment more of a challenge. Self-monitoring with dual-track thinking is helpful in that regard. Once again, it is most important to keep in mind that *clients have the necessary strengths and resources to help themselves.*

12

The Solution-Focused
Approach to Crisis

Crisis in the context of the theory proposed in this book is a point in a living system's drift through life when its structure coupling is in jeopardy. In other words, the survival of a person's life, lifestyle, or relationship is threatened.

However, crisis is generally seen as having the potential for positive change as well as possible disaster. Onnis (1990, p. 43) points out that the word "crisis" is derived from the Greek verb *krino* (I judge or I choose) and therefore suggests choice, or "a moment in which various perspectives and various opportunities present themselves."

DIVERSE RESPONSES TO CRISIS

Fontes (1991) points out that the choices clients make in a crisis depend on their therapist's beliefs. For example, approaches that view crisis and noncrisis situations as totally different (Everstine & Everstine, 1983; Golan, 1978; Meyerson & Glick, 1976; Rapaport, 1962) generally believe that it is the therapist's responsibility to provide structure and direction. Elmer-Dewitt (1989, p. 79) suggests interventions tailormade to particular situations because crises are difficult to categorize exactly. Other models are based on viewing crisis in a series of steps (Caplan, 1964; Rapoport, 1962; Sachs, 1968). Caplan suggests that intervention must be thought of as a reestablishment of a natural homeostatis between people and their environment (Smith, 1978, p. 397). This is reminiscent of structure coupling.

Fontes's own model based on social constructionism suggests that because the truth cannot be determined, the therapist must determine whether it is useful to act as if there is a crisis and employ any of the aforementioned interventions that he or she deems appropriate. However, in such a model the therapist must recognize that he or she is a participant in the coconstruction of the meaning of the crisis and also its possible resolution: "An action taken by a constructivist clinician might in any given case resemble that of another clinician, but the attitude toward the work would probably differ, and I expect a skilled constructivist clinician would perpetrate less violence on clients than a clinician limited to an absolutist view" (p. 66).

This chapter addresses a solution-focused approach to working with cases that are, or may be, in crisis.

WHAT IS CRISIS?

Betty, the client discussed in Chapter 4, was sent for help by her employee assistance program because of sudden crying spells that she felt were out of her control.

A solution-focused colleague shared a story of sitting behind a one-way mirror with a team formulating a summation message when she noticed that her client, a 19-year-old woman, was cutting her thigh with a knife.

A couple brought their daughter to therapy because she had swallowed five Tylenol pills the night before and then called a girl-friend to tell her what she had done. The parents wanted the girl hospitalized.

A therapist is alerted by a client's wife that he is carrying a gun.

What do all these cases have in common?

1. Danger of physical harm to self or other.
2. Danger perceived by someone other than the client (including the therapist) of danger to the client or someone else.
3. Self-perceived lack of control over emotions.

These all constitute emotionally charged situations that challenge therapists to rescue clients. Of course, the idea of rescuing clients is contrary to the position solution-focused therapists generally take, based on the assumption that *clients have the strengths and resources to help themselves* as long as they are aware of their resources. However, as helping professionals our obligation goes beyond theoretical purity; it calls for social responsibility, as well.

THE NEED TO WEAR TWO HATS

The Therapist Hat

When we wear the solution-focused brief therapist's hat we assume that in the course of living human beings run into some situations that are critical, such as illnesses, the death of significant others, hurricanes, blizzards, fires, violence, problematic job situations and relationships, to mention just a few. The meaning particular situations have for a unique individual determines whether we view these experiences as normal events in life or as critical. Once a client and therapist begin to talk about a potentially critical situation, its meaning to the client can change for better or worse depending on the client. As long as the therapist continues to trigger change with the client based on how the client cooperates, he or she can be thought of as still wearing the therapist's hat.

The Social Control Agent Hat

As licensed professionals we are bound by policies and rules developed by the society in which we live (i.e., the government and our professional organizations). These prescriptions for practice were developed to protect our clients from us and from themselves, and also to protect society from our clients. Therefore, when we believe that a conversation with a client who experiences himself, or is experienced by others, as being out of control is creating less safety or control for him and/or others we must put on a social agent hat. Otherwise, if the client should harm him- or herself, or someone else, we would have to account for what we did to prevent the tragic incident. If we cannot, we may lose the right to practice and/or we may be sued.

How to Decide Which Hat to Wear

Wearing two hats can be problematic. For example, take a situation in which a therapist discovers that a client convicted of battery and sent to therapy for anger management acted in a violent manner again after several months of good progress. His wife did not report the act. The therapist is obligated to report the offense to the probation officer, who will have the client arrested again. However, this reporting will probably jeopardize the therapist's relationship with the client and impede the progress that had begun to benefit the client as well as his wife and their children. If the therapist does not report the reoffense, he or she is not only breaking a law but will be held responsible if the wife is seriously harmed in the future.

How, then, does a solution-focused therapist decide which hat to wear, or how to wear both?

Mark Becker of North Central Health Center, Wausau, Wisconsin, contributed the following case example as typical of cases that require a switch in hats.

CASE EXAMPLE: RANDY

Randy, age 14, and his family were referred because of Randy's increasing "blow-ups" at home and at school, consisting of aggressive behavior, destruction of property, and threats of self-harm and suicide.

Randy lived with his mother and two older brothers, ages 16 and 17 in a cramped mobile home. His parents had divorced several years earlier and Dad had little contact with the boys. Randy's brothers were also doing poorly in school.

The therapist started the session by inquiring about exceptions to the current difficulties and about effective deescalating methods but did not get any information. Essentially, everyone felt at the mercy of Randy's "blow-ups."

In an effort to reestablish some confidence and hope, the therapist asked the family how they had been able to cope with the current difficulties. How come things are not worse? Everyone agreed that it was their strong relationship with each other that kept them going. They described various activities that they enjoy together and the mother showed particular pride in the fact that Randy had volunteered at a nursing home.

With the family feeling buoyed by the conversation about their connection with each other, the therapist asked the miracle question and learned that were a miracle to occur Randy would be managing his frustration without "blowing up," making more positive self-statements, attending school successfully, and eliminating self-harm threats. Randy's mother said that in case of a miracle she would complete her high school education and find a better job. One brother's miracle entailed completing high school and entering the military. The whole family wanted a better place to live.

Given the suicidal threats, the therapist had to address safety issues directly and develop a crisis plan for the future. The safety assessment indicated that Randy was not at imminent risk and that no hospitalization was indicated. However, a clear crisis plan was developed with Randy, his family, and school staff.

The summation message highlighted the struggles that had led to this session and noted the family's strong bonds and their goals for the future. A simple suggestion was made for Randy and his family to notice anything that Randy tried to do to avoid a "blow-up," even if it was an insignificant gesture. The therapist also informed the family that he would be talking with Randy's teachers to ask them to be on the lookout for helpful things as well.

Although Randy's mother and the school staff had been invigorated by the new treatment approach, Randy had had another "blow-up" at school and seemed angry during the next session. The therapist told Randy's mother that no one could change Randy, that he could only decide to do that himself.

Two days later Randy kicked the principal at school and had to be removed by the police. He had also been reported to have been physically aggressive with his mother and brothers, thrown the cat against the wall, and wrapped a cord around his neck threatening to kill himself.

When he came to the next session with his mother, Randy was clearly different. He was more depressed but also more agitated. In answer to what happened he said, "I'm a failure in life and I wish I wasn't born." Randy's mother expressed concern about her safety and that of her other sons. She also worried that Randy might follow through on his suicidal threats.

Fear was now added to the hopelessness the family had expressed before. In an effort to assess the need for hospitalization, the therapist asked some scaling questions.

THERAPIST: (to Mom) It sounds like you're both worried about Randy and somewhat frightened of him. If you were to rate your worry on a scale from 0 to 10, with 10 as worried as you can possibly be and 0, not worried at all, where would you say you are today?

MOM: Last night was really scary. Randy has been upset before, but last night was bad. I'd say I'm at about an 8 or 9 right now. He's just been talking about hurting himself so much lately.

THERAPIST: If you were going to rate your present fear of Randy on the same scale, where are you?

MOM: I think what Randy did last night reminded all of us of some of the stuff his dad used to do. When he left, I think we all agreed we didn't want to live like that anymore. Now here we are again. Randy's doing the same stuff.

THERAPIST: So where would you scale your fear today?

MOM: I guess at about an 8 or 9, too.

THERAPIST: Randy, what do you think about what your mom just said?

RANDY: It doesn't make me feel good. I'm a stupid jerk.

THERAPIST: So if you were to rate how worried you are about hurting yourself or others, what would you say?

RANDY: Right now, maybe a 7. But last night I was like a 10. I'm dangerous when I'm mad. I hurt people. I punch and kick.

THERAPIST: It seems like you both agree that this is a scary and dangerous situation.

The therapist gathered some more basic safety information and learned that Randy's suicidal ideations had increased, that he had significant sleep disturbance, increased irritability, and a more pronounced depressed mood. Randy added that he had just learned that he flunked all his classes.

The therapist used another scaling sequence to determine how this episode compared to past episodes. Randy and his mother thought that it was an 8 to 9 compared to a 6 to 7 in the past. He had always been hospitalized when things reached that point, but they said the hospitalization changed little. Hospitalization had only been useful to give everyone a break so they could recharge their batteries. Did their batteries need recharging at this point? Mother repeated her concerns about everyone's safety and Randy indicated that he was "run down."

All questions about what would move the scale down just a little had failed. Randy's mother was unable to describe anything that would make her feel safe at home. The therapist had to put on his social agent hat and recommend hospitalization at this point.

However, solution-focused therapists try to contextualize hospitalization as "a first step to a different future" rather than "a break to recharge." The latter can suggest continuation of the existing behavior rather than change in the future.

THERAPIST: So if we were to look ahead to the day when Randy is ready to leave the hospital, how will we know it has been helpful?

MOM: I would like to know that Randy would have some ways to control his anger when he's upset about something. He always seems to leave before he learns anything new.

THERAPIST: Why is that?

MOM: I start to feel bad about him being away from home. Randy's always begging me to let him come home. He promises he'll change and I guess I want to believe him.

THERAPIST: Yes, it is hard when your child is away from home and homesick. But it sounds like this time you'd like to feel more confident before you bring Randy home. You want to know that he has some new coping skills.

MOM: Yes. I don't think I can let him come right home this time.

THERAPIST: What would be some things that would help you feel more confident that Randy was more prepared to handle things?

MOM: He'd take things more seriously. He'd take responsibility for what he's done instead of blaming someone else or acting like nothing happened.

THERAPIST: How would you know Randy was taking more responsibility?

MOM: He'd stop begging me to come home. He'd apologize for some of his actions and he would be able to tell us how he was going to handle his blow-ups in the future.

THERAPIST: You feel like Randy's going to the hospital could be the first step to a different future if you both do some things differently.

MOM: Right. We both have to change, not just Randy. I have to stick to my guns.

THERAPIST: Randy, what do you think about what Mom is saying? Do you understand where she is coming from?

RANDY: Yeah, but I'm not going to like it. When I first go I want to change, but after I'm there a while, I just want to get out.

THERAPIST: I'm guessing that you're tired of going to the hospital again and again. I also know from our last talk that you care a lot about your family and feel badly about harming them. What do you think it would take for this to be your last trip to the hospital?

RANDY: I have to figure out what to do when I'm mad so this stuff doesn't happen.

THERAPIST: Why do you think that hasn't happened when you went to the hospital before?

RANDY: Because I think more about getting out than about my blow-ups. I know if I work on Mom long enough she'll take me back home.

MOM: I'm telling you now, it's not going to happen this time.

THERAPIST: So the first step to this hospitalization being different is for Randy to not ask about coming home before staff says he's ready. And if he does ask, for you, Mom, to say no.

MOM: It'll be hard, but that's what I have to do.

THERAPIST: So Randy, you said before that you needed to figure out what to do when you get angry. What do you have to do differently this time to come up with these answers while you're in the hospital?

RANDY: I don't like people asking me questions. It gets me angry. But I guess I'm going to have to listen to the questions and figure the other stuff out.

THERAPIST: Even though you don't like it, do you think it will be easier to face the questions if Mom sticks to her guns? If she doesn't let you come home until she feels confident that you've at least started to come up with some answers?

RANDY: I guess so, but I'm not promising that I won't work on her a little.

What made this therapist decide not to recommend hospitalization in the first session but to do so in the subsequent one?

Most solution-focused therapists experienced in working with crisis say that although the safety issue is foremost, they do not address it until the end of the session unless the client is acting out, or threatening to, then and there. Instead, they try to connect, understand, and clarify what everyone in the session thinks and wants, and whether there is the possibility for even a very small change toward the expressed goals. In the first session, Randy's therapist accomplished these steps by listening to the stated problems and asking for exceptions and coping skills. Although no one in the family seemed to have any sense of control over Randy's "blow-ups," the conversation did bring forth the family's positive relationship and a sense of a better future.

Randy's threats of self-harm and aggressive behavior toward others obligated the therapist to assess present safety and develop a crisis plan for the future. The therapist therefore kept his therapist hat on and trusted that the family had the resources to help itself. He had also noted on intake information that there had been previous short hospitalizations but they clearly had not been too helpful. Randy proved not to have a premeditated suicide plan but rather to express his suicidal thoughts impulsively when he felt hopeless. He owned no weapons and there were none in the home. He seemed revolted by the idea of ingesting anything to kill himself for fear of choking or vomiting. He was sleeping and eating fairly normally. The blow-ups had increased in the past few weeks but he seemed motivated to change. Randy appeared eager to participate in the crisis planning and his mother and brothers seemed more hopeful at the end of the session.

The therapist had also noted on intake information that there had been previous short hospitalizations but they clearly had not been helpful, so based on the assessment he kept on his therapist hat and gave the family an appointment for the following week.

When Randy's acting out continued to escalate the therapist had to put on his other hat. After assessing the family's perception of the severity of the present episode compared to past ones he had to ensure Randy's safety and that of others by recommending hospitalization; however, he did so by developing a different context for it from the start.

URGENCY

When lives are at stake, or loss of emotional control, it is natural for clients, their families, the community, and therapists to want relief from the fear as quickly as possible. Clients come to therapy looking to the therapist to make that happen.

The client observed mutilating herself must be stopped immediately even if it takes the police to do it. The client carrying the gun must be convinced to give it to someone for safekeeping, or he must be arrested as quickly as possible. Situations clearly representing imminent danger have to handled expeditiously. Therapists must have the tools to help themselves control their own fears in order to be helpful to others.

Beyond that, however, the most important thing the solution-focused brief therapist can do for clients in crisis is not to identify with their urgency and to be guided by the assumption that *brief therapy goes slowly.* For therapists to succumb to pressure to act quickly (except to prevent harm) can actually be detrimental in the long run because it provides external control rather than promoting internal control that can have a lasting effect. As much as possible, the therapeutic goal for clients who are out of control should be an experience that can help them have more control in the future, in a similar situation.

Dual-track thinking (Chapter 2) that monitors our own internal conversation is a helpful technique for fighting urgency:

Track 1: I'm feeling scared. I'm not sure what to do.

Track 2: What is the client feeling?

Track 1: The client is feeling helpless because she has no control. That's the same way I feel.

Track 2: If I'm scared I can't help her get control. What do I need to get some control?

Track 1: More information from the client about what would make her feel in control. *Clients have the strengths and resources to help themselves.*

LISTENING

When people are fearful and their adrenalin starts pumping they become flooded with emotion that focuses them on action for survival, to fight or to flee. Their attention is more on the figure than on the background. The contrast between crisis/noncrisis becomes exaggerated. The most helpful response by the solution-focused therapist is one that draws attention to a both–and perspective, the shades of gray. This is best accomplished by hearing everything the client says and consciously listening for exceptions and strengths (see Chapter 3). In other words, when therapists open themselves up fully to every aspect of the client's language there is a better chance of finding a response that may trigger some control and hope for the future in the client.

A TIGHT TIME FRAME

Jim Derks (personal communication, November 15, 2000), one of the original developers of SFT, points out the need to establish a "tight time frame" when working with a critical situation.

CASE EXAMPLE: PHILIP

The case of Philip, a 32-year-old single man who was brought to therapy by his brother Pat because of talk about suicide, provides an example of what that means. Pat had become alarmed by Philip's despondency during a phone conversation the night before. Pat knew Philip was unhappy with his work but did not feel qualified to find a more challenging position. However, during that conversation Philip said he had recently gotten two warnings about work performance that he felt were unwarranted, that his relationship with his girlfriend was ending because she was not sure about her feelings for him anymore, and that things had gotten so bad overall that the only solution was to "check out."

After that conversation, Pat went to Philip's house and convinced him to talk to someone about his state of mind. Philip had refused at first but agreed when Pat asked him to do it for the sake of their mother, who had recently gone through chemotherapy for breast cancer and was still feeling weak. Pat then called the hot line of Philip's employee assistance program. After a phone assessment the counselor urged Pat not to leave Philip alone that night and to bring him in the next morning.

THERAPIST: (*Starts by telling Philip he has some information already about the situation.*) Philip, I understand your brother called last night and spoke to the hot line because you were feeling so down and were having some suicidal thoughts.

PHILIP: Yes.

THERAPIST: Are you still having some of those thoughts this morning?

PHILIP: Well . . . umm . . . I . . . I guess so.

THERAPIST: (*Focuses on last night first.*) So, what was going on last night?

PHILIP: It was just the last straw.

THERAPIST: What was?

PHILIP: Terry . . . that's my girlfriend . . . she knows how bad things have been at work for me and now she adds to it by saying she doesn't know how she feels about me (*starts sobbing*).

THERAPIST: That must have been quite a blow. (*Waits quietly while Philip cries for a few minutes.*)

PAT: Hey, Phil, you've got all of us . . . we love you . . . we're here. Mom's going to be all right.

THERAPIST: Is your mom ill?

PAT: She had breast cancer and they've done chemotherapy. She's a fighter. She'll come through.

Philip continued to cry for another few minutes and then started telling his story about what had been going on in his life for the past few months. The therapist did not interrupt or question any details about the story at that time. He just listened and made empathic sounds and gestures. He then refocused the client to the previous night.

THERAPIST: So what made you call your brother last night?

PHILIP: I called about some lottery tickets. We usually go in together with our other brother and buy a whole bunch. It's getting up there now so I wondered when he wanted to get some.

The therapist noted that the client was future oriented, which is a positive sign. He checked out Philip's support system by assessing the health of his relationships with family members and friends. How often do they have contact by phone, personally? He then went back to the tight time frame.

THERAPIST: So what happened during the phone conversation last night about the lottery tickets that made you talk about suicide?

Derks says that it is important to anchor the pain in the immediate past, presupposing that today is different, that is, better: *A small change can lead to bigger changes.*

PHILIP: Well, he said something about Terry going in with us and that just set me off.

THERAPIST: So Pat came over right away when you got so upset.

PHILIP: Yeah.

THERAPIST: And then what happened?

PHILIP: We talked some more . . .

THERAPIST: Did that help?

PHILIP: Yeah. He's always pretty helpful.

THERAPIST: So his coming over made you feel better.

PHILIP: Yeah.

The therapist now attempted to trigger the perceptions that things were different this morning than last night, even if only a small change had occurred. He talked with Pat about whether Philip had any breakfast and established that he ate some cereal. He asked who drove to the session and complimented Philip for letting Pat take care of him by driving. He asked Pat about times when Philip had taken care of him and got some examples. He listened for everything and anything he could reinforce as change from last night. This type of probing does not assume that if the client comes up with positive examples the client is no longer depressed. Rather, it is a small step out of either–or thinking, the beginning of the construction of a solution that may be complex and take time.

THERAPIST: So, Philip, where would you say your stress level is right now compared to last night? [Note that the therapist started talking about "stress level" rather than despondency or suicide.] Put it on a scale from 1 to 10, with 10 as bad as it can get and 1 as good as it can get. [If Philip answers he is still the same or worse, the therapist will have to discuss hospitalization.]

PHILIP: (*Thinks a while.*) I was a 9 last night. I guess I'm more like an 8 now . . . maybe 7.

THERAPIST: Well, realistically you've got a lot of things going on that are disturbing. Is there anything you can think about doing about your work situation that would bring that scale down half a notch today or tomorrow?

PHILIP: I contacted my union rep about those warning yesterday. I have a meeting with him tomorrow. [More future orientation]

THERAPIST: What about the situation with your girlfriend? If a miracle happened tonight and you work up tomorrow morning feeling less hopeless about your relationship what will you be doing differently?

PHILIP: I guess I'd call her.

THERAPIST: What will you say?

PHILIP: I'll tell her I'm angry. This isn't fair. She doesn't tell me what's bothering her. I haven't got a chance that way. I want to talk about this.

THERAPIST: Sounds like a good idea. But let's take one step at a time. How about today, when you leave here? What do you need to keep the stress level down?

The therapist and client continued to talk about how to keep that day and the next day less stressful. They discussed the meeting with the union rep in detail so Philip could anticipate how to respond as much as possible. The therapist made another appointment with Philip to discuss plans for talking with his girlfriend. Arrangements were made for Philip to have dinner with Pat and his family that night.

Evidence of some positive movement does not mean the therapist can ignore the suicidal threats that brought the client in. Therefore, he scaled the degree of Philip's suicidal feelings at this point and found that they were at about a 6. A safety plan was developed that includes Pat and some of the other siblings. The therapist asked Philip to sign a contract that he would not act on any suicidal thoughts without first calling him at an emergency number, which he agreed to.

Derks believes that it is important to ask as many people as possible who know the client to attend the first crisis session. This is not only for the purpose of support but because multiple perspectives about the client and his or her situation offer more information that may trigger an immediate change. The whole idea about a tight time frame is to restrict the focus in order to make a small change more visible and more potent. A panoramic review and search for resources at first can be overwhelming and therefore dangerous.

CONCLUSION

Crisis is a matter of definition that must be clarified by the therapist with the client. The assumption that *clients have strengths and resources to help themselves* and that *a small change can lead to bigger changes* must not be abandoned too hastily; on the other hand, safety must be the first consideration. Everything discussed about SFT in this book so far applies doubly in crisis: careful listening, understanding the client's world view, trying to use language to construct a both–and rather than either–or view, and going as slowly as the situation allows. In SFT it seems most fitting to start out wearing the therapist hat unless a client is totally out of control physically or emotionally. Establishing an emotionally safe climate before exerting control may ultimately make it easier for clients to gain control of themselves. It will also benefit the therapist–client relationship if the client returns for aftercare.

Final Thoughts

Everyone is much more simply human than otherwise.
—HARRY STACK SULLIVAN (1953c, p. 32)

This book, the culmination of over 20 years of thinking about what I do when I talk to clients, is an accumulation, an integration, and a creation of interactions with others. The purpose in writing it was to steer clinicians away from the arbitrary use of technique toward a path they could travel without fear of getting lost. The best outcome from this effort would be that readers are stimulated to think more about why they do what they do when they talk with clients. Facing and explaining the choices we make is a first step on a long road toward mastery. Even the poor choices we make have so much to offer us in the end.

The experience of teaching solution-focused therapy has constantly confirmed for me that every person is unique. Naturally, some people are more sensitive and empathic than others. Everyone may not have the qualities of a master therapist, but we are all human. We know what we need from each other at a basic level without having to say the words. That is why I have emphasized the emotional aspects of therapy along with the technical. I noticed that this combination makes therapeutic skills blossom faster.

The advances from the field of neuroscience that are rapidly enhancing our understanding of human behavior will undoubtedly offer new knowledge and skills to us as psychotherapists in the future. Let us welcome them with an open mind but never forget the importance of humility in our work.

References

Adams, J. F., Piercy, F. P., & Jirhc, J. A. (1991). Effects of solution-focused therapy's "Formula First Session Tasks" on compliance and outcome in family therapy. *Journal of Marital and Family Therapy, 17*(3), 277–291.

Ahlers, C. (1992). Solution-oriented therapy for professionals working with physically impaired clients. *Journal of Systemic Therapies, 11*(3), 53–68.

Alizur, Y. (1996). Involvement, collaboration, and empowerment: A model for consultation with human-service agencies and the development of family oriented care. *Family Process, 35*(2), 191–211.

Andersen, T. (1991). *The reflecting team.* New York: Norton.

Andersen, T. (1995). Reflecting processes; acts of informing and forming: You can borrow my eyes, but you must not take them away from me! In S. Friedman (Ed.), *The reflecting team in action* (pp. 11–37). New York: Guilford Press.

Andersen, T. (1997). Researching client–therapist relationships: A collaborative study for informing therapy. *Journal of Systemic Therapies, 16*(2), 125–134.

Anderson, H. (1997). *Conversation, language, and possibilities: A postmodern approach to therapy.* New York: Basic Books.

Anderson, H., & Goolishian, H. (1986). Systems consultation with agencies dealing with domestic violence. In L. C. Wynn, S. H., McDaniel, & T. T. Weber (Eds.), *Systems consultation: A new perspective for family therapy* (pp. 284–299). New York: Guilford Press.

Bachelor, A., & Horvath, A. (1999). The therapeutic relationship. In M. A. Hubble, B. L. Duncan, & S. D. Miller (Eds.), *The heart and soul of change* (pp. 133–179). Washington, DC: American Psychological Association.

Bachrach, L. L. (1989). Case management: Toward a shared definition. *Hospital and Community Psychiatry, 40*, 883–884.

Barker, P., & Herlache, M. (1997). Expanding the view of treatment with an MPD client and her family. *Journal of Systemic Therapies, 16*(1), 47–59.

Bateson, G. (1979). *Mind and nature: A necessary unity.* New York: Dutton.

Bateson, G., Jackson, D. D., Haley, J., & Weakland, J. H. (1956). Toward a theory of schizophrenia. *Behavioral Science, 1*, 251–264.

Berg, I. K. (1994). *Family-based services: A solution-focused approach.* New York: Norton.

Berg, I. K., & Kelly, S. (2000). *Building solutions in child protective services.* New York: Norton.

215

Berg, I. K., & Miller, S. D. (1992). *Working with the problem drinker: A solution-focused approach.* New York: Norton.

Bergin, A. E., & Lambert, M. J. (1978). The evaluation of therapeutic outcomes. In S. L. Garfield & A. E. Bergin (Eds.), *Handbook of psychotherapy and behavior change: An empirical analysis* (2nd ed., pp. 139–189). New York: Wiley.

Beyebach, M., Morejon, A. R., Palenzuela, D. L., & Rodriguez-Arias, J. L. (1996). Research on the process of solution-focused therapy. In S. D. Miller, M. A. Hubble, & B. L. Duncan (Eds.), *Handbook of solution-focused brief therapy* (pp. 299–335). San Francisco: Jossey-Bass.

Beyebach, M., Rodriguez-Sanchez, M. S., Arribas de Miguel, J., Herrero de Vega, M., Hernandez, C., & Rodriguez-Morejon, A. (2000). Outcome of solution-focused therapy at the University Family Therapy Center. *Journal of Systemic Therapies, 19*(1), 116–129.

Bonjean, M. (1989). Solution-focused psychotherapy with families caring for an Alzheimer patient. In G. Hughston, V. Christopherson, & M. Bonjean (Eds.), *Aging and family therapy: Practitioners perspectives on Golden Pond* (pp. 1–11). New York: Haworth Press.

Bonjean, M. J. (1996). Solution focused brief therapy with older adults and their families, In T. Hargrave & S. Hanna (Eds.), *Between generations* (pp. 1–11). New York: Brunner/Mazel.

Booker, J., & Blymyer, D. (1994). Solution-oriented brief residential treatment with chronic mental patients. *Journal of Systemic Therapies, 13*(4), 53–69.

Bower, G. H. (1981). Mood and memory. *American Psychologist, 36,* 129–148.

Bradshaw, J. (1988) *Healing the shame that binds you.* Deerfield Beach, FL: Health Communications.

Brasher, B., Campbell, T. C., & Moen, D. (1993). Solution oriented recovery. *Journal of Systemic Therapies, 12,* 1–14.

Breunlin, D., & Cade, B. (1981). Intervening in family systems with observer messages. *Journal of Marital and Family Therapy, 7,* 7–46.

Brown-Standridge, M. D. (1989). A paradigm for construction of family therapy tasks. *Family Process, 28*(4), 471–489.

Cade, B., & O'Hanlon, W. H. (1993). *A brief guide to brief therapy.* New York: Norton.

Cantwell, P., & Holmes, S. (1995). Cumulative process: A collaborative approach to systemic supervision. *Journal of Systemic Therapies, 14*(2), 35–47.

Caplan, G. (1964). *Principles of preventive psychiatry.* New York: Basic Books.

Cecchin, G. (1987). Hypothesizing, circularity, and neutrality revisited: An initiation to curiosity. *Family Process, 26*(4), 405–415.

Cecchin, G., Lane, G., & Ray, W. (1992). *Irreverence—A strategy for therapists' survival.* London: Karnac Books.

Cecchin, G., Lane, G., & Ray, W. (1994). *The cybernetics of prejudices in the practice of psychotherapy.* London: Karnac Books.

Chapman, A. H. (1976). *Harry Stack Sullivan: The man and his work.* New York: Putnam's.

Cushman, P. (1995). *Constructing the self, constructing America.* Reading, MA: Addison-Wesley.

Dahl, R., Bathel, D., & Carreon, C. (2000). The use of solution-focused therapy with an elderly population. *Journal of Systemic Therapies, 19*(4), 45–56.

Damasio, A. (1994). *Descartes' error: Emotion, reason, and the human brain.* New York: Putnam's.

Damasio, A. (1999). *The feeling of what happens: Body and emotion in the making of consciousness.* New York: Harcourt Brace.

DeJong, P., & Hopwood, L. E. (1996). Outcome research on treatment conducted at the Brief Family Therapy Center, 1992–1993. In S. D. Miller, M. A. Hubble, & B. L.

Duncan (Eds.), *Handbook of solution-focused brief therapy* (pp. 272–299). San Francisco: Jossey-Bass.

Dell, P. (1982). Family theory and the epistemology of Humberto Maturana. *Family Therapy Networker, 6*(4), 26, 39, 40, 41.

Dell, P. (1985). Understanding Bateson and Maturana: Toward a biological foundation for the social sciences. *Journal of Marital and Family Therapy, 11,* 1–20.

de Shazer, S. (1982). *Patterns of brief family therapy: An ecosystemic approach.* New York: Guilford Press.

de Shazer, S. (1984). The death of resistance. *Family Process, 23,* 79–93.

de Shazer, S. (1985). *Keys to solution in brief therapy.* New York: Norton.

de Shazer, S. (1988). *Clues: Investigating solutions in brief therapy.* New York: Norton.

de Shazer, S. (1991a). *Putting difference to work.* New York: Norton.

de Shazer, S. (1991b). Muddles, bewilderment, and practice theory. *Family Process, 30*(4), 453–459.

de Shazer, S. (1994). *Words were originally magic.* New York: Norton.

de Shazer, S., & Molnar, A. (1984). Four useful interventions in brief family therapy. *Journal of Marital and Family Therapy, 10*(3), 297–304.

Dolan, Y. M. (1991). *Resolving sexual abuse: Solution-focused therapy and Ericksonian hypnosis for adult survivors.* New York: Norton.

Donovan, J. M. (1999). Short-term couple therapy and the principles of brief treatment. In J. M. Donovan (Ed.), *Short-term couple therapy* (pp. 1–12). New York: Guilford Press.

Durrant, M. (1995). *Creative strategies for school problems: Solutions for psychologists and teachers.* New York: Norton.

Efran, J. S., & Lukens, M. D. (1985) The world according to Humberto Maturana. *Family Therapy Networker, 9*(3), 22–29.

Efran, J. S., Lukens, M. D., & Lukens, R. J. (1990). *Language, structure and change: Frameworks for meaning in psychotherapy.* New York: Norton.

Efron, D., & Veenendaal, K. (1993, Spring). Suppose a miracle doesn't happen: The non-miracle option. *Journal of Systemic Therapies,* 11–19.

Ekman, P. (1992). Facial expressions of emotion: new findings, new questions. *Psychological Science, 3,* 34–38.

Elmer-Dewitt, P. (1989, September 25). Time for some fuzzy thinking. *Time,* p. 79.

Erickson, M. (1977). Hypnotic approaches to therapy. *American Journal of Clinical Hypnosis, 20,* 20–35.

Erickson, M. H., & Rossi, E. (1979). *Hypnotherapy: An exploratory casebook.* New York: Irvington.

Erickson, M. H., Rossi, E., & Rossi, E. (1976). *Hypnotic realities.* New York: Irvington.

Everstine, D. S., & Everstine, L. (1983). *People in crisis: Strategic therapeutic interventions.* New York: Brunner/Mazel.

Fisch, R., Weakland, J. H., & Segal, L. (1982). *Tactics of change: Doing therapy briefly.* San Francisco: Jossey-Bass.

Fish, J. M. (1997). Paradox for complainants? Strategic thoughts about solution-focused therapy. *Journal of Systemic Therapies, 16*(3), 266–274.

Fisher, L., Anderson, A., & Jones, J. E. (1981). Types of paradoxical intervention and indications: Contraindications for use in clinical practice. *Family Process, 20*(1), 25–37.

Fontes, L. A. (1991). Constructing crises and crisis intervention theory. *Journal of Strategic and Systemic Therapies, 10*(2), 59–69.

Frankel, A. J., & Gelman, S. R. (1998). *Case management: An introduction to concepts and skills.* Chicago: Lyceum Books.

Frankl, V. E. (1957). *The doctor and the soul: An introduction to logotherapy.* New York: Knopf.

Frankl, V. E. (1960). Paradoxical intention. *American Journal of Psychotherapy, 14,* 520–535.

Fraser, J. S. (1995). Process, problems, and solutions in brief therapy. *Journal of Marital and Family Therapy, 21*(3), 265–281.

Freedman, J., & Combs, G. (1996). *Narrative therapy.* New York: Norton.

Friedlander, M. L., Ellis, M. V., Raymond, L., Siegel, S. M., & Milford, D. (1987). Convergence and divergence in the process of interviewing families. *Psychotherapy, 24,* 570–583.

Friedman, S. (1993, Spring). Does the "miracle question" always create a miracle? *Journal of Systemic Therapies, 75.*

Friedman, S., & Lipchik, E. (1997). A time-effective, solution-focused approach to couple therapy. In J. M. Donovan (Ed.), *Short-term couple therapy* (pp. 325–360). New York: Guilford Press.

Gergen, K. (1982). *Toward transformation in social knowledge.* New York: Springer-Verlag.

Gergen, K. (1991). *The saturated self.* New York: Basic Books.

Gergen, K. (1994). *Realities and relationships: Soundings in social construction.* Cambridge, MA: Harvard University Press.

Gilligan, S. (1997). *The courage to love: Principles and practices of self-relations psychotherapy.* New York/London: Norton.

Gingerich, W. J., de Shazer, S., & Weiner-Davis, M. (1988). Constructing change: A research view of interviewing. In E. Lipchik (Ed.), *Interviewing* (pp. 21–33). Rockville, MD: Aspen.

Gingerich, W. J., & Eisengart, S. (2000). Solution focused brief therapy: A review of the outcome research. *Family Process, 39*(4), 477–498.

Golan, N. (1978). *Treatment in crisis situations.* New York: Free Press.

Goodman, H. (1986). *BRIEFER: An expert system for brief family therapy.* Unpublished master's thesis, University of Wisconsin–Milwaukee.

Goodman, H., Gingerich, W. J., & de Shazer, S. (1989). BRIEFER: An expert system for clinical practice. *Computers in Human Services, 5,* 53–67.

Gottman, J. M., & Levenson, R. W. (1986). Assessing the role of emotion in marriage. *Behavioral Assessment, 8,* 31–48.

Griffith, J. L., & Griffith, M. E. (1994). *The body speaks: Therapeutic dialogues for mind–body problems.* New York: Basic Books.

Haley, J. (1973). *Uncommon therapy: The psychiatric techniques of Milton H. Erickson, M.D.* New York: Grune & Stratton.

Haley, J. (1976). *Problem-solving therapy: New strategies for effective family therapy.* San Francisco: Jossey-Bass.

Harlow, H. F., & Harlow, M. K. (1962). Social deprivation in monkeys. *Scientific American, 207,* 136–146.

Held, B. S. (1996). Solution-focused therapy and the postmodern: A critical analysis. In S. D. Miller, M. A. Hubble, & B. L. Duncan (Eds.), *Handbook of solution-focused brief therapy* (pp. 27–44). San Francisco: Jossey-Bass.

Held, B. S. (2000). To be or not be theoretical: This is the question. *Journal of Systemic Therapies, 19*(1), 35–50.

Hoffman, L. (1981). *Foundations of family therapy: A conceptual framework for systems change.* New York: Basic Books.

Hoffman, L. (1985). Beyond power and control: Toward a "second order" family systems therapy. *Family Systems Medicine, 3,* 381–396.

Hoffman, L. (1990). Constructing realities: An art of lenses. *Family Process, 29*(1), 1–13.

Hoffman, L. (1998). Setting aside the model in family therapy. In M. F. Hoyt (Ed.), *The handbook of constructive therapies: Innovative approaches from leading practitioners* (pp. 100–116). San Francisco: Jossey-Bass.

Horvath, A. O., & Symonds, B. D. (1991). Relation between working alliance and outcome in psychotherapy: A meta-analysis. *Journal of Counseling Psychology, 38,* 139–149.

Hoyt, M., & Friedman, S. (1998) Dilemmas of postmodern practice under managed care and some pragmatics for increasing the likelihood of treatment authorization. *Journal of Systemic Therapies, 17*(5), 12–23.

Hoyt, M. F., & Berg, I. K. (1998). Solution-focused couple therapy: Helping clients construct self-fulfilling realities. In M. F. Hoyt (Ed.), *The handbook of constructive therapies: Innovative approaches from leading practitioners* (pp. 314–341). San Francisco: Jossey-Bass.

Hubble, M. A., Duncan, B. L., & Miller, S. D. (1999) Directing attention to what works. In M. A. Hubble, B. L. Duncan, & S. D. Miller (Eds.), *The heart and soul of change: What works in therapy* (pp. 407–447). Washington, DC: American Psychological Association.

Jackson, D. (1959). Family interaction, family homeostasis, and some implications for conjoint family psychotherapy. In J. Masserman (Ed.), *Individual and familial dynamics* (pp. 122–141). New York: Grune & Stratton.

Jackson, D. (1963). *The sick, the sad, the savage, and the sane.* Unpublished manuscript presented at the annual lecture to the Society of Medical Psychoanalysis and Department of Psychiatry, New York Medical College.

Johnson, M. (1987). *The body in the mind.* Chicago: University of Chicago Press.

Johnson, S. M., & Greenberg, L. S. (1994). Emotion in intimate interactions: A synthesis. In J. S. Johnson & L. S. Greenberg (Eds.), *The heart of the matter: Perspectives on emotion in marital therapy* (pp. 297–323). New York: Brunner/Mazel.

Kanter, J. (1989). Clinical case management: Definitions, principles, components. *Hospital and Community Psychiatry, 40,* 361–368.

Keeney, B. P. (1979). Ecosystemic epistemology: An alternative paradigm for diagnosis. *Family Process, 18,* 117–129.

King, E. (1998). Roles of affect and emotional context in solution-focused therapy. *Journal of Systemic Therapies, 17*(2), 51–65.

Kiser, D. (1988). *A follow-up study conducted at the Brief Family Therapy Center.* Unpublished manuscript.

Kiser, D., & Nunnally, E. (1990). *The relationship between treatment length and goal achievement in solution-focused therapy.* Unpublished manuscript.

Kiser, D. J., Piercy, F. P., & Lipchik, E. (1993). The integration of emotions in solution-focused therapy. *Journal of Marital and Family Therapy, 19*(3), 233–242.

Kleckner, T., Frank, L., Bland, C., Amendt, J., & Bryant, R. du Ree. (1992). The myth of the unfeeling strategic therapist. *Journal of Marital and Family Therapy 18*(1), 41–51.

Kowalski, K. (1987). Overcoming the impact of sexual abuse: A mother's story. *Family Therapy Case Studies, 2*(2), 13–18.

Kowalski, K., & Kral, R. (1989). The geometry of solution: Using the scaling technique. *Family Therapy Case Studies, 4*(1), 59–66.

Kral, R. (1992). Solution-focused brief therapy: Applications in the schools. In M. J. Fine & C. Carlson (Eds.), *The handbook of family–school intervention: Systems perspective* (pp. 330–346). Boston: Allyn & Bacon.

Kreider, J. W. (1998). Solution-focused ideas for briefer therapy for longer-term clients. In M. F. Hoyt (Ed.), *The handbook of constructive therapies: Innovative approaches from leading practitioners* (pp. 341–358). San Francisco: Jossey-Bass.

Lambert, M. J. (1992). Implications of outcome research for psychotherapy integration. In J. C. Norcross & M. R. Goldstein (Eds.), *Handbook of psychotherapy integration* (pp. 94–129). New York: Basic Books.

Lazarus, R. S. (1982). Thoughts on the relations between emotion and cognition. *American Psychologist, 37,* 1010–1019.

LeDoux, J. (1996). *The emotional brain: The mysterious underpinnings of emotional life.* New York: Touchstone.

Lipchik, E. (1988a). Purposeful sequences for beginning the solution-focused interview. In E. Lipchik (Ed.), *Interviewing* (pp. 105–117). Rockville, MD: Aspen.

Lipchik, E. (1988b). Interviewing with a constructive ear. *Dulwich Center Newsletter,* pp. 3–7.

Lipchik, E. (1991). Spouse abuse: Challenging the party line. *Family Therapy Networker, 15,* 59–63.

Lipchik, E. (1993). "Both/and" solutions. In S. Friedman (Ed.), *The new language of change: Constructive collaboration in psychotherapy* (pp. 25–49). New York: Guilford Press.

Lipchik, E. (1994). The rush to be brief. *Family Therapy Networker, 18,* 34–40.

Lipchik, E. (1997). My story about solution-focused brief therapist/client relationships. *Journal of Systemic Therapies, 16*(2), 159–172.

Lipchik, E. (1999). Theoretical and practical thoughts about expanding the solution-focused approach to include emotions. In W. A. Ray & S. de Shazer (Eds.), *Evolving brief therapies: In honor of John H. Weakland* (pp. 157–158). Galena, IL: Geist & Russell.

Lipchik, E., & de Shazer, S. (1986). The purposeful interview. *Journal of Strategic and Systemic Therapies, 5*(1&2), 88–99.

Lipchik, E., & Kubicki, A. D. (1996). Solution-focused domestic violence views: Bridges toward a new reality in couples therapy. In S. D. Miller, M. A. Hubble, & B. L. Duncan (Eds.), *Handbook of solution-focused brief therapy* (pp. 65–98). San Francisco: Jossey-Bass.

Lipchik, E., Sirles, E. A., & Kubicki, A. D. (1997). Multifaceted approaches in spouse abuse treatment. In R. Geffner, S. B. Sorenson, & P. K. Lundberg-Love (Eds.), *Violence and sexual abuse at home: Current issues in spousal battering and child maltreatment* (pp. 131–149). New York/London: Haworth Press.

Lipchik, E., & Vega, D. (1984). A case study from two perspectives. *Journal of Strategic and Systemic Therapies 4,* 27–41.

Ludewig, K. (1992). *Systemische Therapie.* Stuttgart, Germany: Klett-Cotta.

Mandler, G. (1984). *Mind and body: Psychology of emotion and stress.* New York: Norton.

Maturana, H. R. (1988). Reality: The search for objectivity or the question for a compelling argument. *Irish Journal of Psychology, 9,* 25–82.

Maturana, H. R., & Varela, F. J. (Eds.). (1980). *Autopoiesis and cognition: The realization of the living.* Boston: Reidel.

Maturana, H. R., & Varela, F. J. (1987). *The tree of knowledge: The biological roots of human understanding* (Rev. ed.). Boston: Shambhala.

McKeel, A. J. (1996). A clinician's guide to research on solution-focused brief therapy. In S. D. Miller, M. A. Hubble, & B. L. Duncan (Eds.), *Handbook of solution-focused brief therapy* (pp. 251–272). San Francisco: Jossey-Bass.

Metcalf, L. (1995). *Counseling toward solutions: A practical solution-focused program for working with students, teachers and parents.* Englewood Cliffs, NJ: Simon & Schuster.

Metcalf, L., Thomas, F. N., Duncan, B. L., Miller, S. D., & Hubble, M. A. (1996). What works in solution-focused brief therapy: A qualitative analysis of client and therapist perceptions. In S. D. Miller, M. A. Hubble, & B. L. Duncan (Eds.), *Handbook of solution-focused brief therapy* (pp. 335–351). San Francisco: Jossey-Bass.

Meyerson, A. T., & Glick, R. A. (1976). Introduction. In R. A. Glick, A. T. Meyerson, E.

Robbins, & J. A. Talbott (Eds.), *Psychiatric emergencies* (pp. 3–7). New York: Grune & Stratton.

Miller, G., & de Shazer, S. (1998). Have you heard the latest rumor about . . . ? Solution-focused therapy as a rumor. *Family Process, 37*(3), 383–379.

Miller, S. D. (1994). The solution conspiracy: A mystery in three installments. *Journal of Systemic Therapies, 13*(1), 18–38.

Minuchin, S. (1974). *Families and family therapy.* Cambridge, MA: Harvard University Press.

Molnar, A., & de Shazer, S. (1987). Solution focused therapy: Toward the identification of therapeutic tasks. *Journal of Marital and Family Therapy, 13*(4), 349–358.

Molnar, A., & Lindquist, B. (1989). *Changing problem behavior in schools.* San Francisco: Jossey-Bass.

Moxley, D. P. (1989). *The practice of case management.* Newbury Park, CA: Sage.

Murphy, J. J. (1996). Solution-focused brief therapy in the school. In S. D. Miller, M. A. Hubble, & B. L. Duncan (Eds.), *Handbook of solution-focused brief therapy* (pp. 185–204). San Francisco: Jossey-Bass.

Nau, D. S., & Shilts, L. (2000). When to use the miracle question: Clues from a qualitative study of four SFBT practitioners. *Journal of Systemic Therapies, 19*(1), 129–135.

Nichols, M. P., & Schwartz, R. C. (1995). *Family therapy* (3rd ed.). Boston: Allyn & Bacon.

Norum, D. (2000). The family has the solution. *Journal of Systemic Therapies, 19*(1), 3–16.

Nunnally, E., de Shazer, S., Lipchik, E., & Berg, I. (1986). A study of change: Therapeutic theory in process. In D. E. Efron (Ed.), *Journeys: Expansion of the strategic-systemic therapies* (pp. 77–97). New York: Brunner/Mazel.

Nylund, D., & Corsiglia, V. (1994). Becoming solution-forced in brief therapy: Remembering something important we already knew. *Journal of Systemic Therapies, 13*(1), 5–12.

O'Hanlon, W. H., & Weiner-Davis, M. (1989). *In search of solutions.* New York: Norton.

Onnis, L. (1990). A systemic approach to the concept of crisis. *Journal of Strategic and Systemic Therapies, 9*(2), 43–54.

Orlinsky, D., Grawe, K., & Parks, B. (1994). Process and outcome in psychotherapy. In A. E. Bergin & S. E. Garfield (Eds.), *Handbook of psychotherapy and behavior change* (4th ed., pp. 270–375). New York: Wiley.

Panksepp, J. (1998). *Affective neuroscience: The foundation of human and animal emotion.* New York: Oxford University Press.

Papp, P. (1980). The Greek chorus and other techniques of paradoxical therapy. *Family Process, 19*, 45–57.

Parry, A. (1984). Maturanation in Milan. *Journal of Systemic and Strategic Therapies, 3*(1), 35–43.

Patterson, C. H. (1984). Empathy, warmth, and genuineness in psychotherapy: A review of reviews. *Psychotherapy, 21*, 431–438.

Penn, P. (1982). Circular questioning. *Family Process, 21*(3), 267–280.

Penn, P. (1985). Feed-forward: Future questions, future maps. *Family Process, 24*(3), 299–311.

Pinsof, W. M. (1995). *Integrative problem centered therapy.* New York: Basic Books.

Raiff, N. R., & Shore, B. K. (1993). *Advanced case management: New strategies for the nineties.* Newbury Park, CA: Sage.

Rapaport, L. (1962). The state of crisis: Some theoretical considerations. *Social Service Review, 36*, 112–117.

Ray, W. (2000). Don D. Jackson—A re-introduction. *Journal of Systemic Therapies, 19*(2), 1–7.

Rober, P. (1999). The therapist's inner conversation in family therapy practice: Some ideas about the self of the therapist, therapeutic impasse, and the process of reflection. *Family Process, 38*(2), 209–229.

Rohrbaugh, M., Tennen, H., Press, S., & White, L. (1981). Compliance, defiance, and therapeutic paradox: Guidelines for strategic use of paradoxical interventions. *American Journal of Orthopsychiatry, 51*(3), 454–467.

Rosenberg, B. (2000). Mandated clients and solution-focused therapy: "It's not my miracle." *Journal of Systemic Therapies 19*(1), 90–100.

Sachs, V. K. (1968). Crisis intervention. *Public Welfare, 26,* 112–117.

Schmidt, G., & Trenkle, B. (1985). An integration of Ericksonian techniques with concepts of family therapy. In J. K. Zeig (Ed.), *Ericksonian psychotherapy: Vol. II. Clinical applications* (pp. 132–155). New York: Brunner/Mazel.

Selekman, M. D. (1997). *Solution-focused therapy with children: Harnessing family strengths for systemic change.* New York: Guilford Press.

Selvini Palazzoli, M., Cecchin, G., Prata, G., & Boscolo, L. (1978). *Paradox and counterparadox: A new model in the therapy of the family in schizophrenic transaction.* New York: Jason Aronson.

Shaffer, J., & Lindstrom, C. (1989) *How to raise an adopted child.* New York: Crown.

Shields, C. G., Sprenkle, D. H., & Constantine, J. A. (1991). Anatomy of an initial interview: The importance of joining and structuring skills. *American Journal of Family Therapy, 19,* 3–18.

Simon, D. (1996). Crafting consciousness through form: Solution-focused therapy as a spiritual path. In S. D. Miller, M. A. Hubble, & B. L. Duncan (Eds.), *Handbook of solution-focused brief therapy* (pp. 44–65). San Francisco: Jossey-Bass.

Simon, R. (1985). Structure is destiny: An interview with Humberto Maturana. *Family Therapy Networker, 9*(3), 32–46.

Smith, L. L. (1978). A review of crisis intervention theory. *Social Casework, 2,* 396–405.

Spitz, R. A. (1951). Hospitalism: An inquiry into the genesis of psychiatric conditions in early childhood. In *The psychoanalytic study of the child* (Vol. 6, pp. 255–278). New York: International Universities Press.

Sprenkle, D. H., Blow, A. J., & Dickey, M. H. (1999). Common factors and other nontechnique variables in marriage and family therapy. In M. A. Hubble, B. L. Duncan, & S. D. Miller (Eds.), *The heart and soul of change: What works in therapy* (pp. 329–361). Washington, DC: American Psychological Association.

Stanton, M., Duncan, B., & Todd, T. C. (1981). Engaging resistant families in treatment. *Family Process, 20*(3), 261.

Sullivan, H. S. (1953a). *The collected works of Harry Stack Sullivan: Vol. 1. Book 2. Conceptions of modern psychiatry.* New York: Norton.

Sullivan, H. S. (1953b). *The collected works of Harry Stack Sullivan: Vol. 1. Book 1. The interpersonal theory of psychiatry.* New York: Norton.

Sullivan, H. S. (1953c). *The interpersonal theory of psychiatry.* New York: Norton.

Sullivan, H. S. (1953d). *The psychiatric interview.* New York: Norton.

Sullivan, H. S. (1956). *Clinical studies in psychiatry.* New York: Norton.

Todd, T. C. (1981). Paradoxical prescriptions: Applications of consistent paradox using a strategic team. *Journal of Strategic and Systemic Therapies, 1*(1), 28–44.

Tohn, S. L., & Oshlag, J. A. (1996). Solution-focused therapy with mandated clients: Cooperating with the uncooperative. In S. D. Miller, M. A. Hubble, & B. L. Duncan (Eds.), *Handbook of solution-focused brief therapy* (pp. 152–184). San Francisco: Jossey-Bass.

Tomm, K. (1984). One perspective on the Milan systemic approach: Part 1. Overview of development, theory and practice. *Journal of Marital and Family Therapy, 10*(2), 113–127.

Tomm, K. (1987a). Interventive interviewing: Part I. Strategizing as a fourth guideline for the therapist. *Family Process, 26,* 3–13.

Tomm, K. (1987b). Interventive interviewing: Part II. Reflexive questioning as a means to enable self-healing. *Family Process, 26,* 167–184.

Tucker, N. L., Stith, S. M., Howell, L. W., McCollum, E. E., & Rosen, K. H. (2000). Meta-dialogues in domestic violence—focused couples treatment. *Journal of Systemic Therapies, 19*(4), 45–56.

Turnell, A., & Edwards, S. (1999). *Signs of safety: A solution and safety oriented approach to child protection casework.* New York: Norton.

Turnell, A., & Lipchik, E. (1999). The role of empathy in brief therapy: The overlooked but vital context. *Australian and New Zealand Journal of Family Therapy, 20*(4), 177–182.

Varela, F. J. (1989). Reflections on the circulation of concepts between a biology of cognition and systemic family therapy. *Family Process, 28*(1), 15–25.

von Foerster, H. (1991). *Observing systems.* Seaside, CA: Intersystems.

Walter, J. L., & Peller, J. E. (1992). *Becoming solution-focused in brief therapy.* New York: Brunner/Mazel.

Walter, J. L., & Peller, J. E. (1994). "On track" in solution-focused brief therapy. In M. F. Hoyt (Ed.), *Constructive therapies* (pp. 111–126). New York: Guilford Press.

Walter, J. L., & Peller, J. E. (1996). Rethinking our assumptions: Assuming anew in a postmodern world. In S. D. Miller, M. A. Hubble, & B. L. Duncan (Eds.), *Handbook of solution-focused brief therapy* (pp. 9–27). San Francisco: Jossey-Bass.

Watzlawick, P. (Ed.). (1984). *The invented reality.* New York: Norton.

Watzlawick, P., & Weakland, J. (1977). *The interactional view.* New York: Norton.

Watzlawick, P., Weakland, J., & Fisch, R. (1974). *Change: Principals of problem formation and problem resolution.* New York: Norton.

Weiner-Davis, M., de Shazer, W., & Gingerich, W. J. (1987). Building on pretreatment change to construct the therapeutic solution: An exploratory study. *Journal of Marital and Family Therapy, 13,* 359–363.

White, M. (1995). *Re-authoring lives: Interviews and essays.* Adelaide, South Australia: Dulwich Centre.

White, M., & Epston, D. (1990). *Narrative means to therapeutic ends.* New York: Norton.

Wynn, L. C., McDaniel, S. H., & Weber, T. T. (1986). *Systems consultation: A new perspective for family therapy.* New York: Guilford Press.

Zajonc, R. B. (1984). On the primacy of affect. *American Psychologist, 39,* 117–123.

Index